DR. SEBI SMOOTHIES CLEANSE BOOK

THE APPROVED DETOX GUIDE WITH 100 DELICIOUS ALKALINE SMOOTHIE RECIPES FOR NATURAL LIVER CLEANSING, FAST WEIGHT LOSS, AND HEALING YOUR BODY

Tasha Dixon

Table of Contents

Introduction

Why fruits and vegetables are so important

One of the most important benefits of eating more fruits and vegetables is that they are low in calories but high in nutrients. But there's much more to it than just that. Vegetables can be a good source of many minerals, such as magnesium, potassium, and iron. They also contain B vitamins and fiber. Fruits provide the body with potassium, calcium, thiamin (vitamin B1), riboflavin (B2), niacin (B3), pantothenic acid (B5), folate (B9), and vitamin C.

In addition to this, fruits and vegetables are good sources of fiber. Fiber can help you feel full after eating a meal so that you don't consume excess calories. Soluble fiber, which dissolves in the water and can help lower blood cholesterol levels by trapping bile acids before they get absorbed into the body.

The Importance of Clean Raw Juice

The benefits of the extracted juices of fruits and vegetables prepared with fresh vegetables and in season are known to all: they are foods rich in vitamins, minerals, and trace elements, antioxidants, and enzymes in quantity, depending on the mix can have energizing properties, draining, detox or anti-aging. These are the good reasons to include extracted juices in the daily diet. The water contained in the extracted juices, moreover, is of very good quality, the best water you can find, really healthy for our well-being.

Drinking fruit and vegetable juices is important because it allows us to consume large quantities of nutrients while avoiding fiber which, although very useful and necessary for the cleaning and health of the intestine, has no nutritional value. The presence of fiber makes digestion long and laborious, whereas the extracted juice is digested almost directly by making available to the body, in a very short time, all the nutritive substances.

Another advantage is given by the fact that eventual pesticides remain inside the fiber: in this way, in case the vegetable or the fruit chosen were not from organic farming, the extracted juice would still be a "healthy" juice even from this point of view.

Therefore, live juices, highly moisturizing, are particularly indicated in slimming diets and for the depuration of the body, keeping intact the heritage of nutrients such as vitamins, salts, and enzymes which are highly beneficial for the body and its balance.

Top sign and symptoms you need Dr. Sebi's Detox smoothies.

If you find yourself in some or many of these symptoms, it is a sign that your body is urgently in need of purifying, and you can do it through the intake of precious substances coming from fresh juices and centrifuges.

1. Difficulty in concentrating
2. Constipation
3. Headache
4. Gas and bloating
5. Joint pain such as aches in knees and back
6. Heartburn
7. Mood swings
8. Nervousness and confusion
9. Unusual hair loss or flaking of the skin like in cases of psoriasis or alopecia.

Dr. Sebi's Detox cleanses program is suitable for all ages including post-menopausal women over 60 years old to children over 10 years old (with parental supervision).

The best time to start this new program is first thing in the morning after waking up and before eating anything else.

Dr. Sebi Approve Smoothie Cleanse Detox

In the past, I have always been a skeptic of "fasting" or "cleansing". Then I started experimenting with the one by Dr. Sebi. All I can tell you is that it was a cathartic and revelatory experience, as my body was so intoxicated that I didn't realize it, and when I started the cleanse, I had some heavy reactions at first due to the detoxification, but that slowly, day by day, gave way to a renewed feeling of well-being, lightness, strength.

I hadn't done it for weight loss, but for the overall sense of well-being, you get from cleansing your entire system and eliminating those constant cravings for carbs and sugar, one of the detoxing effects, so it's really worth a try.

Dr. Sebi's smoothies fit perfectly into a balanced dietary context and give that extra boost to detoxification, which should be experienced at least every season change.

Dr. Sebi's smoothies are like eating your favorite food at a restaurant without a sense of guilt. They are easy to make and once you find the one you like best, it becomes your favorite meal. I have no problem going to work on a liquid diet, you can't even say I'm fasting. I drink my smoothie religiously every morning and never crave carbs or sugar. It has really changed my life for the better since discovering this way of nutrition.

What happens by drinking Dr. Sebi's smoothies:

What I really like about Dr. Sebi's smoothies is that they are all natural and contain no artificial sweeteners or preservatives. Dr. Sebi's smoothies are packed with nutrients with little to no calories and the high fiber content makes them enjoyable. I started drinking one every morning for breakfast. The taste and texture of the smoothie gives a nice start to the day.

The first time I tried the smoothie, I was blown away by the way it made me feel. It tasted delicious, and after finishing the bottle, I felt like I could run a marathon. My energy level was boosted to the max and my hunger pangs went away for hours and every day. This is a great way to reduce excess calorie consumption and lose weight at the same time.

I always bring my smoothies with me, for breakfast, lunch, and dinner. No matter where I am, I don't get hungry until the evening, and then when I do get hungry, all it takes is a little snack that just helps you stick to the plan.

I highly recommend trying the detox tea. Sure, it's not as tasty as smoothies, but it did a good job of cleansing my system and I felt better after drinking it than any other detox tea or drink I have ever taken before. I discovered some great flavors! It has a mild flavor but cleanses you well and gives you the energy you need for an active day. It's also excellent for mornings after a night in the town where you know you've been drinking and eating more than is good for you.

I have to give full credit to Dr. Sebi for creating a truly effective system that actually works. This stuff is amazing, and I can't tell you how much better I feel without being overweight! When it comes to down in losing weight, there are only two things: hard work, and dedication. You have to be focused and plan ahead to stay on track. But you can see the results, big time. I am dedicated to losing weight and continue to be so with each day that goes by.

How It Works

A Quick Overview of Smoothie Cleanse

A very common question is: does a smoothie help you to lose weight? And the answer is yes! It can be a powerful and fantastic tool, but only when you know how to use it correctly.

Green smoothies are salvation for fading beauty. They help our body to fully detox for weight loss. And it's not only a delicious drink but it's also rich in nutrients that rejuvenate the skin, slow down the aging process, and make your hair healthy and shiny again.

The following questions will help decide if you should consider this type of diet:

- Don't think about your weight, pay attention to your body fat percentage – is it normal?
- Do you feel tired, even after you had a good rest?
- Do you suddenly crave something sweet during the day?
- Do you dull-looking hair, skin, and nails?

Even one "yes" is enough to think about your health and think about a detox cleanse diet. If you are determined to change your life with green smoothies, then here are some steps to follow for a successful start and the best results:

No More Excess Body Fat and Chronic Diseases

What green smoothies can help your body do is get rid of excess fat, making your life much better without it. Nutrients are responsible for regulating blood insulin levels in your body. When blood insulin's concentration is higher than normal, more fat is stored inside the body. It can increase the risks of dangerous diseases as renal impairment, heart disease, diabetes, and even several types of cancer, among others. That's why you should control your amount of visceral body fat.

Limit the Toxic Exposure on Your Body

Green smoothies are a great source of natural nutrients that will make your body and immune system much stronger and reduce the inflammatory process. As the source of essential elements for our body, a green smoothie includes natural sugars, minerals, and fiber. A smoothie will help you to be more energetic during the day, thanks to the more efficient processing of its energy sources.

In addition, one of the most important features is the reduction of exposure to toxins and sugar cravings, thanks to the large presence of chlorophyll, a very precious substance. By increasing the intake of nutritious and satiating smoothies, there will be no room for other unnecessary foods, especially junk food. It means it will become easy to steer clear of processed food, and you'll do so unconsciously, thanks to the cancellation of sugar cravings, and satiety. You'll be surprised at how your body will no longer seek out fast-food items if you were used to them.

We must consider toxic exposure as a problem as it causes food intolerances and allergies. Our body will be protected from such disease only if we enrich our daily diet with essential nutrients and reduce our intake of unhealthy sugars, fats, and preservatives.

Refresh Yourself

With a green smoothie, you will not only improve your body and immune system but also refresh your beauty. All the smoothie nutrients will make your hair glow and shine again, and your skin will look healthy and fresh. It will help you to stay hydrated longer and reduce sagging.

Always remember what you eat has a direct effect on your skin and hair. If you often eat junk food, you will notice that your skin and hair become dull-looking, unhealthy, and dehydrated.

Functions of the Liver

The liver is an important organ in the abdominal cavity. The main functions of the liver are to produce bile, which helps break down fats in food and so aids digestion; to store sugar (glycogen) for energy production; to make certain proteins needed by the body, and to detoxify poisonous substances such as alcohol or drug medications.

The liver is often referred to by its more specific names — "the chemical factory," "the digestive system's garbage can" or "nature's biological sewage treatment plant." Indeed, when your liver malfunctions, your bowels may back up with undigested food that will need removal by enemas — usually a sign that you should seek medical care. The liver is also a major filtering system, which is why it's also often referred to as "the body's natural filter."

It weighs about three pounds and has a reddish-brown color. It's located on the right side of your abdomen (abdomen), just below the rib cage. You can feel the upper part of your liver behind your right rib cage by pressing with a finger about an inch and a half above the bottom of your breastbone (sternum).

The liver has three main functions:

- To make and store glycogen (sugar) for energy.

- To produce bile, which helps break down fats.

- And to detoxify poisonous substances such as alcohol or drug medications.

A liver that's healthy, working properly, is clear of fat and toxins — a lean liver with a healthy coloration will have a light green color. When the liver becomes weak or diseased, it turns yellow or deep purple, or black in color. Inflammation of the liver also causes your skin to turn yellowish-red and your eyes to become puffy (jaundiced).

The liver is shaped like a melon in cross-section. The main sections are the hepatic lobe, or right lobe, and the cystic lobe, or left lobe. The lobes join at the porta hepatis, which is located on top of the pancreas. The cystic lobes are like tiny islands of cells in a sea of clear water — they contain and protect the tiny bile ducts that drain into a central vein. The membrane that surrounds each island is called a sinusoid or hepatic canalicular membrane — these sine waves, which look much like water ripples on a pond when viewed through a microscope, arrange themselves into pairs called bile ductulus (one for each ductile).

Toxins Effect on the Liver

A healthy liver is crucial to the body's health. When a person is exposed to toxins, the body typically tries to process and flush them out of the system. However, when heavy toxic exposure begins limiting an individual's ability to get rid of these toxins naturally through their liver, they can lead to cancer and other serious illnesses. The liver is the large glandular organ that functions in the metabolism, detoxification, and transportation of substances through the body. When it comes to toxins, there are two primary ways that they can be removed from the system. The liver can either be processed or then excreted through bile, or it can be stored in fat tissue or muscle tissues in extreme cases.

Heavy metals are one of the largest contributors to this type of burden on the liver. Lead poisoning can greatly affect the central nervous system, with early symptoms being a loss of appetite, irritability, and sleep disturbances. Western society is loaded with these toxins through contaminated foods, air, and water. Heavy metals have also been found to be part of the reason for cancer in many cases.

Importance of Liver Cleansing

As one of your major organs, it's important to keep it healthy to maintain good health. Now will explore what liver cleansing entails and why you should care about its wellbeing!

Liver cleansing may seem like some strange new trend or fad diet to most people (it's not). In fact, cultures around the world have relied on this practice for centuries. Liver cleansing is any type of cleansing that helps to remove potentially toxic and unhealthy material from the liver. There are essentially two types of cleanses: "Liver Flushes" and "Liver Cleanses." Liver Flushes are conducted with water or another liquid while Liver Cleanses are usually conducted with herbs, organic fruits, vegetables, and juices.

Why I Need to Drink Cleanse Smoothies

These are some of many amazing benefits of a liver cleanse:

- Rid the body of toxins

- Shed excess weight
- Improve mood
- Remove liver stones
- Increase energy
- Feel more alive and confident
- Age gracefully and look more youthful
- Cleanse your body

Tips on Maintaining Optimal Liver Health

Taking Care of Your Liver Right Now May Prevent Certain Health Problems in the Future

1. Avoid smoking, it not only affects your liver but also puts you at risk for several other diseases. The chemicals in tobacco can damage your arteries, making them narrow and forcing your blood pressure to go up. Secondhand smoke has the same effect. The unhealthier your current lifestyle is, the longer it'll take you to adopt healthy living habits.

2. Avoid alcohol, it's well-known that heavy drinking raises blood pressure. Men, especially those over 65, should not take more than one drink a day, and women should take still less. The older you get, also, the less you should drink.

3. Drink enough spring water at least 1 Liter of spring water daily is one of the easiest ways to maintaining a healthy functioning liver. Water helps to flush out toxins that have accumulated. Natural spring water also contains m minerals that replenish the body and are absorbed by the liver. If you find it difficult to take that much water a day, you can try infused water with a quarter teaspoon of key lime juice.

4. Follow the Dr. Sebi Nutrition Guide Eating, such as having a period of only alkaline electric vegan foods, is the best way to a good liver Health all year round.

If you have any interest in your gut health, you've probably considered or at least heard of the benefits of cleansing. A holistic and healthy digestive system might not seem like it would be important for your overall well-being, but it is! It turns out that the gut is one of the most intricate and influential parts of our body. It does so many things that we often don't even realize — from regulating inflammation to optimizing hormone production, all the way down to providing essential nutrients. With a healthy gut, we can avoid unpleasant symptoms such as bloating, diarrhea, or constipation.

A Self-Reported Diet "Non-Starter"

Many of us have tried to follow a diet in order to lose weight or maintain good health. Most people think that eating less and exercising make up their diet plan — and that is true for the most part. Often, however, along the way we replace good, nutritious foods with unhealthy (and often sugary) substitutes. The result is a diet that only works to curb our hunger and frustration while leaving us unfulfilled. I would describe this tendency as a "non-starter."

Diets that are non-starters are hard to sustain and ensure effective weight loss. As such, people who make it their goal to lose weight do it by lowering their caloric intake, sometimes even limiting themselves to around 1000 calories per day. However, the diet does not provide long-term benefits — in fact, it has been shown to lead to long-term health problems such as heart disease (Henriques). Carbs should be limited (due to their high glycemic index) in order to prevent blood sugar swings, while fat should only be taken in moderation.

You see, all foods contain macronutrients: carbohydrates (CHOs), which provide energy; fat (FATs), which provide fat-soluble vitamins such as A, D, E, and K; and protein (PRIs), which provide amino acids. Together, these macros contribute towards the total nutritional value of food (Trottier). But what about the micronutrients? They are contained largely in vegetables, fruits, and greens, and are incredibly essential building blocks for health. Not only do they lift the performance of the entire body, but we couldn't live without them.

Understanding the Meaning of Alkaline

The term alkaline refers to a substance that produces a neutral pH (or basic) when dissolved in water. This includes substances such as baking soda and potash. Alkaline are compounds that have an alkaline ion H+ or OH-. As it turns out, many foods are either acidic or alkaline — depending on what they contain and how our body can break them down.

The scale of acidity or alkalinity is measured on a pH scale. Each number on the pH scale represents a factor of ten. For example, a solution that measures 3 is ten times more acid than a solution that measures 4. An acid will lower the pH of a solution. A base will raise the pH of a solution.

At room temperature, water is neutral; it doesn't change the volume of any object (the water doesn't expand or contract). But all substances have different natures and react differently to different conditions. Water can be split into oxygen and hydrogen atoms, with an equal number of protons and electrons in each atom. This is called electrolysis, or an alkaline solution. An acid will release hydrogen ions (H+) and oxygen ions (. O2-) in water, which lowers the pH of a solution.

The discharge of H+ is related to the dissociation constant, which is the equilibrium constant for the reaction. The greater the value of the equilibrium constant, the greater will be the release of hydrogen ions in water. The most common way to measure this is by using a pH meter/pH indicator paper.

Importance of Balance pH in the Body

Alkaline Blood and the Role of pH

Dr. Sebi's African Bio-Mineral Balance methodology introduced me to the concept that an acidic body supports the proliferation of disease, and an alkaline body protects against disease. The issue is a bit more complex, which gave people who wanted to be divisive ammunition to attack his methodology. More specifically acidic blood supports the proliferation of disease.

Acid and alkaline are the opposite sides of the pH scale. The scale for pH ranges from 0 pH to 14 pH. 0 pH represents the highest acidic level, and 14 pH represents the highest alkaline level. 7.0 pH is neutral. Though different areas of the body are acidic it is very important to eat alkaline foods to maintain a blood pH of around 7.4. The pH of the blood is the reference point for homeostasis or optimal functioning of the organs in the body.

The body works diligently to keep the blood in a slightly alkaline state near a pH of 7.4 to support homeostasis and health. The pH stands for "potential hydrogen" and has the ability of molecules to attract hydrogen ions. Too many hydrogen ions floating around the bloodstream make the blood acidic and interferes with the proper oxygenation of cells in the body. Eating meat, dairy, processed foods, and even highly hybridized starchy plant foods acidify the blood because of their molecule structure. They also lack vital minerals, vitamins, and phytonutrients the body needs to properly perform metabolic functions.

Health Problems Due to Acidity on the Body

Health problems due to acidity on the body are becoming more and more prevalent. Most people around the world have begun to notice that they are suffering from many health-related problems such as blood pressure, headaches, depression, and heart problems. Studies show that the main cause of this is the acidic nature of their body.

The intake of food is one way in which you can reduce your acidity levels. Foods like fruits, vegetables, legumes, and nuts can help lower your pH level as they have an alkalizing effect on the body. An overabundance of processed foods will have a different effect therefore it's important to reduce or stop eating these types of foods if you want to live a healthier life with less illness.

Another way to reduce acidity levels is by drinking alkaline water. It has been proven that adding magnesium to your water can help reduce the acidity in the body.

When we eat food, many of the nutrients have an alkalizing effect on our bodies. It's recommended that you drink 10 glasses of water and one glass of fresh juice per day as these drinks will help keep your body alkaline. Alkaline foods such as cucumbers, green salads, and raw nuts can also be eaten to help you reach an alkaline pH level.

When we are ill, some people suffer from a highly acidic state. Pain relief, sleep, and relaxation can help you reduce the acidity in your body. Alkalize with herbs such as valerian root to help you fall asleep.

Alkaline foods will also help you maintain a healthier mood. Try to eat more green vegetables such as spinach, lettuce, and celery because they are alkalizing and will also give your body the minerals it needs to keep healthy. You should also drink water because this is a way for the body to excrete alkaline levels from the body.

Why Fruit Vegetable Smoothies Keep you Healthy and Vibrant

Healthy eating is important, and the argument over which foods are healthier is never-ending.

Fruit can be healthful because it contains a variety of nutrients like vitamins A, C, and E, potassium, fiber, and antioxidants to help protect cells from damage caused by free radicals. It can also be an effective tool for weight management because consuming whole fruits gives you a sense of fullness that avoids snacking on high-calorie snacks like chocolate or cookies without the guilt that often accompanies these indulgent foods.

The fiber in fruit also helps curb appetite by encouraging the production of a hormone called cholecystokinin that causes the feeling of fullness. Whenever you eat fruits, cholecystokinin is released into your bloodstream, and this stimulates your brain to send a message to your stomach to tell it to stop eating.

The fiber found in fruits also helps prevent deficiencies and constipation because it stimulates the production of a substance known as butyrate. Butyrate can help maintain normal intestinal function, relieve irregular bowel movements, and thereby increase regularity so that people who have been suffering from constipation can benefit from eating fruit.

It's a well-known fact that vegetables contain essential nutrients, such as calcium, potassium, and vitamins A, C, E, and K. Vegetables are also low in calories so they can be consumed to boost metabolism and increase your energy level. They are also incredibly good for the body because they can help relieve the symptoms of conditions like osteoporosis because they contain vitamin K. Vitamin K can also help reduce your risk of fractures by strengthening bones and teeth.

Vegetables are rich in antioxidants like beta-carotene and lutein that have been studied for their ability to protect against certain diseases including age-related macular degeneration (AMD). It is a disease that can cause pain and vision loss in people over 65, and many studies have indicated that beta-carotene was shown to be very effective in helping prevent the disease. In addition, lutein is a nutrient that helps maintain eye health because it promotes cell growth and prevents harmful free radicals from impairing vision or causing early blindness.

Finally, vegetables are very good for your body because they can reduce inflammation, reduce cholesterol and prevent cancer by slowing the growth of cells associated with certain cancers.

The bottom line is that fruit vegetable smoothies should maintain healthy pH basic because they are high in calories so they stimulate metabolism. Also, they contain fiber which can help control appetite and promote regular bowel movements. Also, fiber is a powerful antioxidant that can help prevent constipation and reduce high cholesterol.

Healthy Guidelines for Preventing Cancer

The best way to ensure a healthy diet is to eat a variety of foods from all the major food groups each day. This can be done by including plenty of fresh fruits and vegetables in your diet. These foods are especially important because they contain powerful antioxidants, minerals, and vitamins that promote good health. It is really a good idea to limit unhealthy fats, sugar, and salt. This can be done by eating less processed foods and limiting consumption of foods that is high in fat such as butter, cheese, and fatty meats. Avoiding or limiting the intake of sugary foods and drinks like sodas and pastries is also a good idea.

People that are concerned with their health should be especially mindful about keeping the sodium (salt) in their diet to a minimum because this substance has been linked to high blood pressure and other health problems. It is important to eat whole grains like brown rice, whole wheat bread, oatmeal, and quinoa because they can lower the risk of heart disease by reducing LDL (bad) cholesterol levels in the body. Regular exercise that involves strength training along with daily physical activity will help people maintain their health by boosting their metabolism and strengthening their muscles.

People even need to protect themselves against the health hazards of unhealthy job exposures. These include strong chemical solvents, pesticides, ammonia, formaldehyde, and carbon monoxide. People who work with these types of chemicals should do the following:

Conduct an initial risk assessment to identify possible problems that are linked to exposure to chemical solvents and other dangerous substances. Take precautions against exposure to these substances by using proper gloves, masks, or goggles when working with chemicals. Work in a well-ventilated area if possible because smoking can expose people to more harmful toxins through their lungs. Make certain that chemical storage areas are well-ventilated and kept at a safe distance from the workplace.

The best way to reduce exposure to potentially toxic products is to work in a well-ventilated area, don protective clothing, such as gloves or masks, and avoid touching your skin with chemical-soaked gloves or other materials.

What is Electric Food Diet

Electric nutrition is a diet based on the use of live foods, rich in an electric charge due to the presence of biophotons, so entirely vegetable. This raises the vibrational level of the body, thanks to the presence of energetic particles contained in the vegetables themselves, which are thus transferred into the body through their intake.

Dr. Sebi created his dietary pathways starting with only the live and raw food groups, virtually excluding the rest of the food groups. He encouraged patients to consume more foods that approximate a natural vegan diet, such as naturally grown vegetables and fruits, and even whole grains. His line of thinking was that live, raw foods are electrical, meaning they give an electrical charge and fight food waste and acids produced in the body.

Dr. Sebi compiled his list of foods that he called the 'Electric Food List,' and considered it the core of his diet.

Electric, Acid and Alkaline.

Electric Food — Acid and Alkaline some foods and drinks change from acidic to alkaline once they are metabolized. This essentially makes them alkaline-based, as once they are digested, they become alkaline. One of the most common foods in this category is citrus fruits, which contain ascorbic acid.

Citrus Fruits

Citrus fruits may be often avoided as they are often considered acidic and sour to taste. Once they are fully digested, they effectively become alkaline in the body, with the results of increasing the pH balance to a more basic or alkaline environment. Fruits that fit into this category include lime, lemon, oranges, mandarins, tangerines, and grapefruit.

Tomatoes

Tomatoes are another example of a fruit that becomes rich in alkaline once consumed. They are naturally acidic, and like citrus fruits, may be avoided due to their sour and sometimes strong taste. Tomatoes are best consumed in a raw state when they are digested quickly and increase the alkaline levels in the blood. When they are stewed, baked, or otherwise cooked, tomatoes increase acidity, though are still very nutritious. If you enjoy tomatoes or cooked varieties are a regular part of your diet, incorporate both raw and cooked versions. For example, if you create pasta dishes, stew some tomatoes, and add some raw slices or cherry tomatoes as a topping to gain their benefits.

Kombucha

Drinks Kombucha is an acidic beverage that is comprised of fermented ingredients. It is typically created with a tea base (green or black tea), with added sugar for the fermentation process to form healthy bacterial cultures. There are many varieties of kombucha and recipes for flavoring and fermentation techniques. Kombucha drinks are growing in popularity in grocery stores and restaurants, though they were once considered a rare treat in upscale eateries and shops. They are available in many flavors and contain a longer shelf life than other fermented foods, such as yogurt, kimchi, and sauerkraut. Why is kombucha beneficial for an alkaline diet? Although it is an acidic beverage, once metabolized, it becomes alkaline in the body. It is beneficial for gut health and aiding in the digestion process, which is due to the role of healthy bacteria, which also prevents infectious diseases and conditions, many of which originate in the gut. The healthy bacteria act as a barrier or protection in the stomach during the digestion process, which keeps acidic levels low to moderate. Kombucha is also high in antioxidants, which is a good defense against cancer, diabetes, and other conditions (for treatment and prevention), which is why this drink is beneficial as part of an alkaline diet.

Pineapples

Many people will avoid pineapples because they can taste sour and cause irritation initially, though they are high in nutrients and alkalinize in the body once consumed. The benefits of pineapples include improving gut health, similarly, to fermented foods, such as yogurt and kombucha. Pineapples also reduce bloating and inflammation, which is caused by a lot of chronic and autoimmune conditions. Joint pain, arthritis, and other conditions that impact the bones and joints can be improved by the amount of vitamin C and antioxidants in pineapples. Vitamin C improves immunity function, which is beneficial for good health in general. If you exercise regularly and include weight or powerlifting as a part of your workout, eating pineapples and fruits high in vitamin C, fiber, and alkaline (once digested) can help your muscles recover quickly.

Apple Cider Vinegar

There are a lot of health benefits of adding apple cider vinegar to your diet, even in small amounts such as a tablespoon or two each day. This is made by mixing fermented apples with yeast and bacteria. Due to the acetic acid levels contained in it, many people avoid it altogether, as it has a pungent taste that is difficult to swallow. Diluting with water or lemon juice is one way to offset the strong taste, as well as adding to a balsamic dressing or another condiment. The benefits of apple cider vinegar work well with an alkaline diet for the following reasons: Apple cider vinegar benefits insulin sensitivity and keeps blood sugar levels normal. While not conclusive, this effect may decrease the likelihood of developing type 2 diabetes. Taken after a meal, can help with the digestive process and curb overeating, which can promote weight loss and management. It's best to consume with water or diluted with a similar drink such as tea or sparkling water to prevent the effects of the acetic acid on tooth enamel and the burning sensation on the mouth and throat if used regularly.

Foods Allowed on the Electric Food Diet

Fructose in Fruits

If you look at the natural development of humankind and food gathering, fruits would have been the easiest food to gather. Fruits didn't need to be prepared, and you could walk up to a tree, pick a piece of fruit, and start eating. Raw, green vegetation was as easy to gather for consumption, but cooking it would have been a bit more time-consuming. Root vegetables and legumes would have been easy to harvest but would have taken the most time to prepare. Acquiring meat for consumption would have taken the most time and would have the most dangerous. From an acquisition standpoint, fruits would have logically been the bulk of the food consumed. Fruits also happened to be loaded with natural fructose that was digested quickly to support the body with quickly accessed energy for its fight-or-flight response in natural environments. Fructose from industrial processing is nothing like the fructose found naturally in fruit. Deprived of fiber, vitamins and minerals, it becomes an empty substance, raising blood sugar and acidification levels in the body. Avoid.

High-Fructose Corn Syrup

Fructose in fruits was naturally packaged by God/the Source of Life/Nature to support a variety of functions in the body. The fiber, fructose, phytonutrients, and other compounds worked together in a way that created synergy and was supportive of bodily functions. High-fructose corn syrup (HFCS) was made only to be useful to the food company. Since HFCS was not packaged with components that controlled its absorption into the bloodstream, HFCS enters the bloodstream and abnormally spikes the blood sugar level. Absolutely avoid.

Refined e Complex Carbs

Refined carbohydrates give to all carbohydrates a bad reputation. Complex carbs are starches and fiber, and refined complex carbs are starches with the fiber removed. The refining process not only removes fiber but also removes most of the food's vitamins, minerals, phytonutrients, and healthy oils. Bread, pasta, cereal, candy, pastries, cakes, cookies, and pies made from enriched and bleach flours are all examples of refined complex carbs.

Complex Carbs and Simple Carbs

Natural complex carbs, grains, and legumes are digested more slowly, and go through the whole glucose-conversion process and contribute to weight gain. Though they have beneficial properties consuming them should be a minimal part of the diet. Both simple carbs and complex are converted to glucose for energy and are stored as glycogen in the liver and muscles. After glycogen storage becomes full in the muscles and liver, excess glucose is converted to triglycerides and is stored in fat cells. Consuming processed additive sugars is problematic because they are not packaged with fiber and nutrients that control their digestion.

Key Rules of Electric Food Diet

The key rules of Dr. Sebi's Electric Food Diet are:

1. Drink more water than you normally would. If you are not used to drinking a lot of water, start drinking a glass of water every two hours until it becomes a habit. You should drink two liters of water a day, preferably natural spring water.

2. Rubber and plastic are toxic materials. Don't take water (or food) from a disposable container where you find remnants or traces of toxic toxins but prefer glass containers.
3. No alcohol, no animal products, no hybrid foods, and no dairy.
4. Eat plenty of vegetables and fruits and get your daily dose of exercise.
5. Don't skip any meals because it will lead to lower blood sugar levels which could prove dangerous. Remember that your body needs the energy from food to function properly.
6. You should not eat any food within two hours of exercise, or it may cause inflammation.
7. Do your exercise in the form of walking, swimming, or biking.
8. Don't use the microwave, which kills food.
9. Don't consume fruit without seeds or fruit in cans.

Smoothies colors are not a fashion

Every day increase the number of "juice bars", places where it is possible to taste many elixirs of wellness such as smoothies, shakes, milkshakes, and centrifuges. It is easy to confuse these denominations, but each of these beverages has specific characteristics. All of them have in common the presence of fruit as the main ingredient. While the blended is more liquid because it is diluted with ice and milk, smoothie instead is much more dense and creamy. Centrifugate instead is a real concentrate of vitamins and mineral salts obtained by centrifuging fruits and vegetables. The extractor contained in the special machines used for centrifuges is capable of separating the juice from the pulp and the peel. Often centrifuges are also called extracts.

Smoothie has become very popular because it is a source of many nutrients such as vitamins and antioxidant properties. Very appreciated at breakfast and at snack time, they are fresh thanks to the presence of ice that keeps them cold but not frozen.

Nutritionists are in favor of smoothies because they respect the rule of five portions of fruits and vegetables per day without the risk of swelling the belly or irritating the bowel. In order to enjoy all the beneficial properties of fruits and vegetables, it is necessary to use seasonal and fresh fruits. The warning is to consume them as soon as they are prepared because the beneficial properties of vitamins are altered with time and during storage in the fridge.

Smoothies are very striking for their bright and gaudy colors. They contain no artificial coloring. The color is created due to the mix of fruits and vegetables and the presence of anthocyanins and pigments.

Each smoothie color is associated with a specific beneficial effect:

- Red: obtained from a mix of strawberries, cherries, turnips, beets promotes the good functioning of the cardiovascular system and fights free radicals;
- Yellow: obtained from citrus fruits, pineapple, carrots. It has an anti-inflammatory power and prevents cellular aging;
- Green: thanks to the contribution of asparagus, mint, basil, rocket, kiwi, avocado has an antioxidant power;
- Purple: a tasty mix of blueberries, red berries, blackberries, figs, and radicchio, it is anti-inflammatory and increases immune defenses.

What You Need to Get Started

Getting Started

During detox cleanse, the body and most importantly, the digestive tract shuts down and this allows the body to focus more on healing because it's no longer using energy to aid and digestion. The amount of time that you cleanse helps a lot in the healing process, so the longer the cleanse, the better the results — but it is not the only factor for good results. It's very important to cleanse at least once per year for 7 days consuming an alkaline diet. However, Dr. Sebi recommends detoxing for 12 days on smoothies, juice, or raw food.

How to Make a Good Natural Smoothie

A common misconception is that fruit and vegetable smoothies are only for healthy people. This couldn't be further from the truth! Everyone — including you — can benefit from drinking a juice or blended drink every day. These drinks can make you feel lighter, cleaner, and have more energy. But not all juices and blends are made equal — some brands contain up to 80% sugar!

Now you might be thinking "that's too much sugar!" And yeah, it's true that this amount of sugar might not be a great way to start your day if you're trying to lose weight or eat better (especially if the rest of your diet is high in refined carbs!). You see, store-bought juices and smoothies are often loaded with sugar, even if they say "100% natural" or "organic." And this is a shame because it means that people with a sweet tooth are choosing over-sweetened juices and smoothies instead of eating fresh fruit.

Without getting too technical, let me explain why store-bought juice and smoothies tend to be sugary. Many brands of juice include added sugar in the form of high fructose corn syrup (HFCS), which is a highly refined starch made from genetically modified corn. HFCS is cheap and easy to use, but it also contains very few vitamins and minerals compared to real fruit.

Now some people prefer the taste of hydrogenated oils (Trans fats), which are formed when liquid vegetable oil is put through high-pressure processing techniques. Tran's fats (hydrogenated oils) are cunningly better tasting than natural fats because they stay liquid at room temperature — you won't notice when you drink a smoothie that has one tablespoon of Tran's fat in it.

Several brands of juices and smoothies use "natural" sweeteners like honey, agave syrup, or maple syrup. These sweeteners are known to be high in fructose and cause the body to absorb them more quickly. Is it a coincidence that recent studies have found that children with high levels of fructose in their blood there are more likely to have obesity, type 2 diabetes, and metabolic theory?

If you want to enjoy healthy fruit smoothies without all the sugar, you'll need a way to get real fruit into your diet and detoxify your system at the same time. So how do you know which fruit is actually good for your health? First of all, you'll need to find a source that has all the vitamins and minerals you need to keep your body running smoothly. Remember that nature-designed fruits with all their various nutrients to work together — combining fruits in a smoothie helps you get a great balance of vitamins and minerals. This is especially important if you're eating lots of fresh produce while on the juice cleanse diet.

How to Get the Right Herbs

A lot of people asked what is the best herbs to get are. There are things to consider when choosing herbs for your kitchen. I've put together some information on how to get the right ones and different ways you can use them in your cooking.

Some people like using fresh herbs, while others prefer dry herbs because they last longer. I think it all depends on the kind of herbs you use in cooking. Most people prefer to have fresh herbs, but they are actually harder to find than dried herbs. If you want fresh herbs you need to grow them yourself or buy them at a local shop, farmer's market or if they are seasonal. The best time to get them is around the end of summer when they are still in season and at their freshest.

Dried herbs are easier to find and store. You can buy dried herbs in the spice section of most supermarkets or in health food stores. They'll usually come in small bottles — get your hands on the containers that come with shaker tops so you can shake them into your cooking easily. When buying dried herbs, it is important to check if they are organic. If you don't, you'll be adding all kinds of pesticides and chemicals into your cooking as well. No one wants to do that.

What to Expect During the Smoothie Detox?

During the detox there are several reactions in the body due to detoxification, namely the elimination of toxins in circulation. You may experience sensations such as:

- Cold and Flu symptoms
- Changes in Bowel movements
- Fatigue and Low Energy
- Difficulty sleeping
- Itching
- Headaches
- Muscle aches and pains
- Acne. Rashes and breakouts
- Mucus expels (catarrh, etc.)
- Lower blood pressure

These symptoms are only temporary and usually resolve after the first one to two weeks.

How to Break Your Smoothie Detox Fast

If you're doing a detox period of just smoothies, centrifuges, herbal teas or water, start by slowly reintroducing solids. You can start by introducing solids such as high water content fruits. These include watermelon, apples, and berries. Later, you can proceed to introducing softer solids such as bananas and avocados. After that, you can incorporate vegetables, following by whole grains. Continue to drink at least 2 liters of spring water daily.

Tips to Motivate You to Get Started

Smoothie Cleanse: tips and advice

If you want to do cleanse, you should be ready for the food and energy fluctuation. A cleanse diet will change your lifestyle, especially you're eating habits. You might feel hunger, headaches, and changes in energy levels while you get used to detox changes.

Don't be afraid to experiment. You don't have to drink only one green smoothie during the diet. Find new recipes and mix different fruit and vegetables to get the best for you. As a result, you won't get bored and will enjoy your smoothies.

Make a smoothie schedule. It's a good habit to have systematic eating, specifically while you on a smoothie cleanse diet. Start with your favorite vegetable smoothie in the morning.

Weight loss and cleansing aren't the same things. The real purpose of a detox diet is to reduce the number of toxins in your body and weight loss is a side effect. This diet even changes our taste buds. It means you will want less junk food and more healthy food.

Listening to your body while doing a detox cleanse. You shouldn't feel bad and suffer during the diet. Watch how your body reacts, have a good rest, if you are extra hungry — get some healthy snacks like fresh vegetables with hummus or something similar, if you have a headache — try to drink more water.

Try to comfort your body! It might be that you feel really horrible on the first or second day of detoxing. It means you have to stop your detox for a little break and wait for the right time to cleanse your body.

Stay hydrated! It's important not only for any diet but and for a healthy lifestyle too. While you cleanse your body, you need to release the toxins from the body, and the water is the best helper! It will improve the elimination process and prevent dehydration, which is especially dangerous while you are on a detox or cleanse diet. Try to drink about 2-3 liters each day during cleansing.

Sleep well during the diet. Your body is working hard, so you need to have extra rest. It's better to sleep at least 8 hours at night and take a short nap during the day if you feel tired.

Don't be upset if something doesn't go as planned. It's not a reason to stop or give up, get back in the game, and go on your cleanse. It's all right if you have missed a meal or take a day off, especially if you need it. Just keep moving!

Avoid any stress and let your mind have a rest too. Try not to overload your schedule with commitments or appointments, give yourself time to relax and do what you like.

The Detox Smoothie Food List Guide

So, you're finally ready to give your body a much-needed break from all the junk food, processed cookies, refined sugar. Good for you! But before you dive into yet another diet that will have you counting calories and feeling deprived 24/7, take a look at this Detox Smoothie Food List Guide. From avocado to leafy greens, it's got everything your body needs for its post-holiday detox.

Don't be too hard on yourself — I know how hard it is to resist the temptation of an ice cream sandwich on a hot day (trust me). Your cravings will subside, I promise.

When you're done reading this guide, you can print out our detox smoothie food list and take it with you as you go grocery shopping! You'll want to be prepared for your next health kick.

Avocado

This superfood is packed with nutrients like vitamin E, potassium, and B-6 that are great for your heart! Also good for repairing damaged skin and hair. Potassium helps prevent high blood pressure and muscle cramps.

Yogurt

We all know that yogurt is great for digestion, but did you also know that it contains probiotics (good bacteria) that help boost your immune system? Yogurt also has vitamin B12 which helps increase energy levels.

Beets

Beets are incredible detoxifiers because they have the ability to remove contaminants from our body and they also help reduce the amount of cholesterol produced by metabolizing fat, according to Prevention. Don't believe me? Try them yourself!

Chia Seeds

Chia is the best source of omega-3 fatty acids, which are known to reduce cholesterol and may lower the risk for heart disease. Omega-3s also help with muscle growth and repair.

Cauliflower (Raw or Cooked)

This cruciferous veggie is rich in vitamins C, K, folate, and manganese-all essential nutrients for our health. It's also a good source of fiber that helps fight off some types of cancer and lowers cholesterol.

Leafy Greens (Lettuce, Spinach, Kale)

You got to get your greens in! They contain a powerful antioxidant called glutathione that helps fight free radicals in the body. Free radicals can damage our cells, which can lead to cancer and heart disease. Glutathione is the perfect anti-aging antidote. Leafy greens are also great detoxifiers due to their high levels of antioxidants and vitamins. It also contains fiber that helps keep you full longer.

Pineapple

Pineapple is one of the richest in bromelain, an enzyme that aids in digestion and may help treat inflammation, arthritis, and respiratory problems like asthma.

Kiwi

Kiwifruit is also good for digestion - and also for intestine - it contains fiber that helps keep you feel full longer. Get your fill of vitamin C!

Grapefruit

Also rich in vitamin C, grapefruit contains bromelain which is a natural enzyme that helps digestive problems. It boosts the immune system and also helps prevent diabetes.

Honey

Honey is so good for you! It's loaded with about 100 different vitamins, minerals, antioxidants, and enzymes that make it one of the healthiest foods that are known to man, it is also great for weight loss because it has a low glycemic index, so meaning it doesn't spike your blood sugar levels as much as white sugar does.

Oatmeal

Oatmeal is also an amazing source of fiber and is great for your heart! It reduces the risk for heart disease because it lowers cholesterol. Also, the soluble fiber in oatmeal helps with blood sugar control for people with type 2 diabetes.

Banana

Bananas are excellent mood boosters because they contain tryptophan — an organic compound that can reduce stress and promote a good night's sleep, according to Dr. Oz. Also good for reducing muscle soreness caused by exercise, much like ibuprofen but without the side effects. Plus, bananas are rich in potassium!

Coconut Water

Did you know coconut water is the most hydrating of any natural beverage? Studies have shown that it helps lower blood pressure and is rich in electrolytes, which can help reduce inflammation!

Spirulina (or Chlorella)

Both are great sources of protein that will keep you full longer. Both are also rich in chlorophyll which gives them their green color. It is a powerful antioxidant that can fight free radicals in your body!

Cucumber

Cucumbers are rich in vitamin B6, which is essential for the metabolism of fat into energy and important for brain function and nerve metabolism.

Organic fruits and vegetables

Fruits, vegetables, nuts, seeds, whole grains, spices, and flavorings are the foods that strengthen the immune system. These foods in fact are precious sources of vitamins (A, B, C, and E) and minerals such as zinc that, as demonstrated by several scientific studies, are essential to strengthen our immune system. Vitamin C, specifically, plays a role of fundamental importance to face infections. In fact, it reduces up to 40% of the harmful action of free radicals on white blood cells and enhances the activity of lymphocytes.

In order to meet the daily requirement of Vitamin C, it is necessary to take about 60-100 mg, a quantity that we can easily find in two oranges or four kiwis. Vitamin C also has a protective function, so it is good to take the recommended daily dose not only in case of ongoing disease but daily, as a form of prevention.

Fruits and vegetables are also very important to ensure the correct intake of carotenoids, the protectors of tissues, and mucous membranes, including those of bronchi and lungs. The vegetables richest in vitamins and minerals useful to defend the immune system are: lemons, kiwi, strawberries, blackcurrants, red peppers, cabbage, avocado, almonds, walnuts, barley, rice, spelt; among spices and condiments we find: turmeric, hot pepper, garlic, onion, parsley, mint, thyme, and oregano. In order to ensure the supply of all these precious substances, we must choose products from organic farming.

Organic farming is based on a method of cultivation that excludes the use of fertilizers, pesticides, herbicides, chemical preservatives of synthesis but uses only substances of natural origin.

Fruit and vegetables from organic farming are 100% natural, it does not contain residues of synthetic chemical products and genetically modified organisms (GMO). In addition, many scientific studies have shown that the products of organic farming have a higher concentration of nutrients, such as vitamins, minerals, and antioxidants.

Choosing organic fruits and vegetables means giving preference to foods grown without the use of pesticides and chemical substances that are harmful to both human health and the environment. Organic fruit and vegetables are naturally tastier and healthier because the methods of cultivation follow the changing of the seasons in a natural way: therefore, eating an organic vegetable, perhaps at km 0, is a much more satisfying experience than eating an imported vegetable, both in organoleptic terms and for our health. Giving preference to organic products is more satisfying and, according to some scientific studies, it would be even better because organic products would contain a higher amount of antioxidants than non-organic ones.

Recipes

Electric Food Smoothies

The red velvet

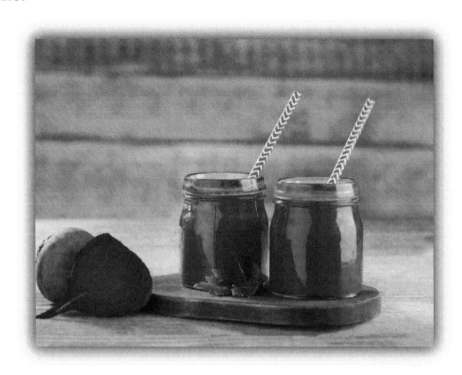

Both are nutrient powerhouses. Pomelos contain 600% of your daily requirement of vitamin C, high in fiber, and helps with circulation. Beets, help with digestion, detox the liver and kidneys, and are high in iron.

> ➢ **Preparation time:** 10 minutes
> ➢ **Servings:** 2

Ingredients:

- 1 medium-sized beet
- 2 large pomelos

Directions:

1. Cut up the beet. Peel and segment the pomelos.
2. Juice them in your Omega juicer.

Blood Orange Chili

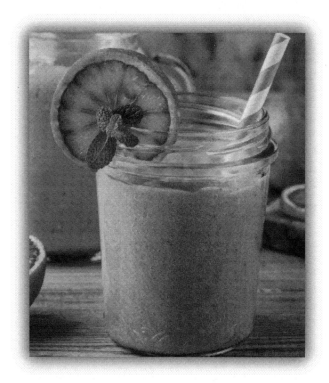

Chilies contain a very powerful anti-inflammatory called capsaicin. Blood oranges contain a phytonutrient called anthocyanins that fights inflammation. Be careful because this is spicy.

- ➢ **Preparation time:** 12 minutes
- ➢ **Servings:** 1

Ingredients:

- 6 blood oranges
- 2 serrano chilies
- Agave nectar (optional)

Directions:

1. Peel the oranges. Slice the chilies in a half and remove the seeds.
2. Gradually press the ingredients in your Omega juicer.
3. Add agave to sweeten if desired.

Blueberry Green Juice

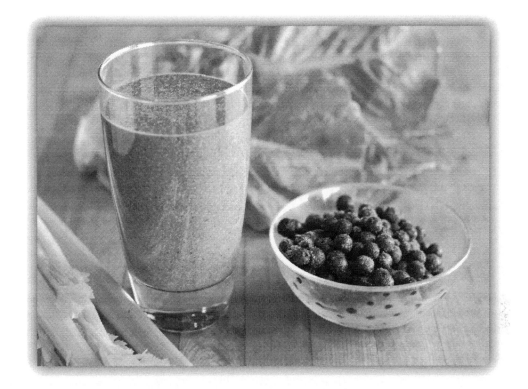

Blueberries are packed with antioxidants that help your overall health. They also contain anti-inflammatory compounds. Spinach is high in vitamin K which boosts memory.

Preparation time: 5 minutes

Cooking time: 5 minutes

Servings: 1

Ingredients:

- 2 cups fresh blueberries
- 2 cups fresh spinach leaves
- 2 Fuji apples

Directions:

1. Cut the apples and remove the seeds. Slice the spinach for about half an inch.
2. Feed the Omega chute alternately with fruits and greens.

Dill-Rightful Glow

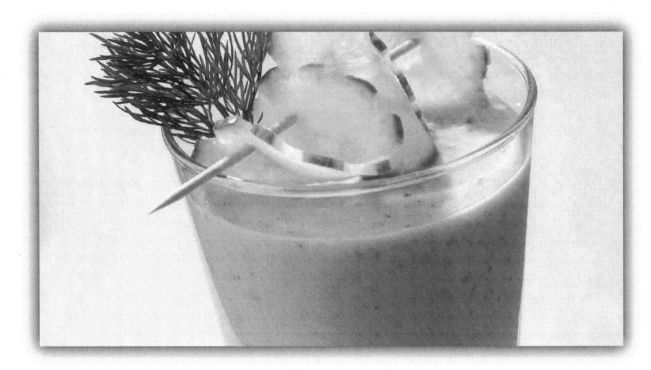

The carrots are packed with antioxidant-rich vitamins A&C. The lemon is alkalizing and will help balance your ph. Dill is mineral-rich, and its essential oil helps to inhibit bacterial growth.

- ➢ **Preparation time:** 7 minutes
- ➢ **Servings:** 2

Ingredients:

- 1 apple
- 1 lemon
- 4 carrots
- 1 head celery
- 1 bunch dill

Directions:

1. Cut the apple and remove the seeds. Peel the lemon. Slice the carrots, celery, and dill.
2. Juice the ingredients in your Omega juicer. Press the dill in between fruits.

Full Spectrum Juice

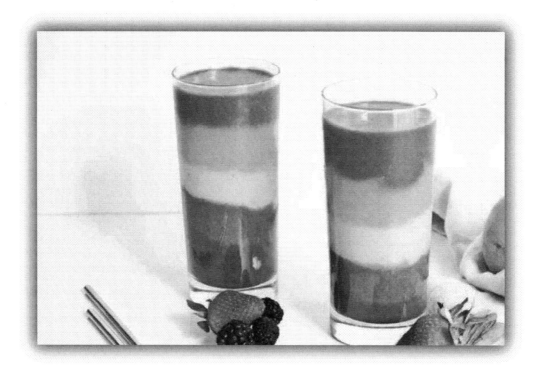

Spinach contains a ton of vitamins, minerals, antioxidants, and phytonutrients. It helps with inflammation, cancer prevention, detoxification, and heart health. Acai and blueberries have anti-inflammatory, anti-microbial, and antibacterial compounds. Strawberry are hydrating and will help remove toxins and help the cells function better. Pineapple is high in vitamin C and is alkalizing.

> ➤ **Preparation time:** 15 minutes
> ➤ **Servings:** 4

Ingredients:

- 1/2 glass of frozen raspberries
- 1/2 glass of frozen strawberries
- 1/2 glass of frozen peeled oranges
- 1/2 glass of frozen mango pulp
- 1/2 glass of pineapple
- 1/2 glass frozen spinach
- 1/4 cup frozen blackberries

- 1/4 cup frozen blueberries
- 5 sliced frozen bananas
- 1 sachet of frozen acai
- 2 glasses of coconut water

Directions:

1. Step 1: Blend ingredients according to color

2. Place the frozen fruit, on a baking sheet, separated by color.

3. You can start by blending the red-colored fruit. Place the strawberries, raspberries, and 1/4 cup of coconut water in the blender bowl. Blend well until the ingredients are combined and then transfer the red smoothie to a bowl.

4. Then switch to the orange color, put the mango, 1/2 banana, and oranges in the blender, then pour 1/4 cup of coconut water and blend well. At this point, as with the previous smoothie, pour the orange smoothie into another bowl.

5. It's time for the yellow-colored ingredients. Put the recommended portion of pineapple, 1 frozen banana, and 1/4 cup of coconut water in the blender, then blend well and transfer the yellow smoothie to a bowl or cup.

6. It's the green color's turn, so place 1 sliced banana, frozen spinach, and 1/4 cup of coconut water in the blender. Turn on the blender and as soon as it's ready, pour the green smoothie into another bowl.

7. You are almost done, make the purple smoothie by putting the blueberries, blackberries, acai sachet, and again 1/4 cup of coconut water in the blender and blend until smooth, then pour the smoothie into a cup, forming layers, and serve the wonderful smoothie to your guests.

Cleansing Smoothie Detox

Peachy Hemp Seed Smoothie

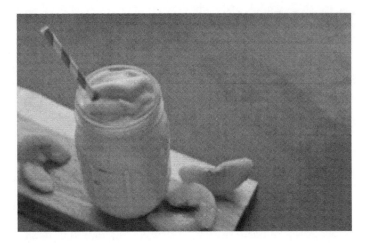

> ➤ **Preparation time:** 5 minutes
> ➤ **Servings:** 2

Ingredients:

- 2 burro bananas, peeled
- 2 tablespoons walnut butter, homemade
- 1 cup peach slices
- 1 tablespoon hemp seeds
- 2 cups spring water

Directions:

1. Plug in a high-speed food processor or blender and add all the ingredients to its jar.
2. Cover the blender jar then pulse for 40 to 60 seconds until smooth.
3. Divide the drink between two glasses and then serve.

The 3 Ingredient Green Smoothie

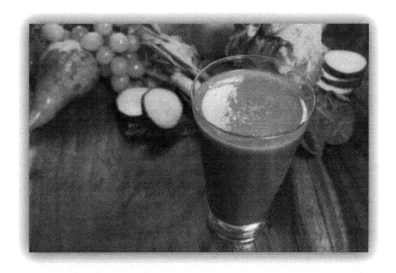

- ➢ **Preparation time:** 5 minutes
- ➢ **Servings:** 2

Ingredients:

- 2 burro bananas, peeled
- ½ cup lettuce
- 1 cup spring water
- 2 cups orange juice, fresh

Directions:

1. Plug in a high-speed food processor or blender and add all the ingredients to its jar.
2. Cover the blender jar and then pulse for 40 to 60 seconds until smooth.
3. Divide the drink between two glasses and then serve.

Dandelion Green Smoothie

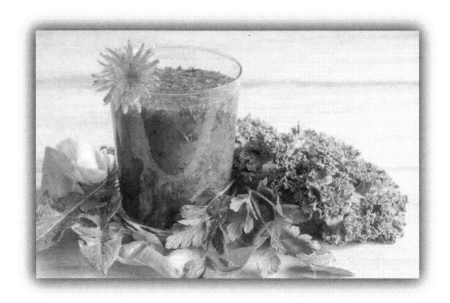

Preparation time: 5 minutes

Cooking time: 0 minute

Servings: 1

Ingredients:

- ½ cup dandelion greens
- ½ of cucumber, deseeded
- ½ apple, cored, deseeded
- ½ burro banana, peeled
- ½ teaspoon Bromide Plus Powder (Optional)

Directions:

1. Plug in a high-speed food processor or blender and add all the ingredients to its jar.
2. Cover the blender jar and then pulse for 40 to 60 seconds until smooth.
3. Divide the drink between two glasses and then serve.

Tamarind and Cucumber Drink

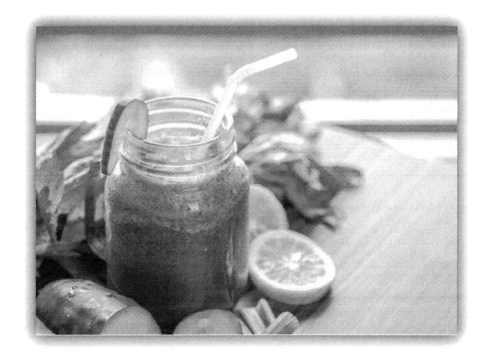

> **Preparation time:** 5 minutes
> **Servings:** 1

Ingredients:

- 1 cup Dr. Sebi's Herbal Tea
- ½ tablespoon tamarind pulp
- ½ cucumber, deseeded
- 1-ounce arugula
- ½ key lime, juiced
- ¼ teaspoon salt
- 1/8 teaspoon cayenne pepper

Directions:

1. Plug in a high-speed food processor or blender and add all the ingredients to its jar.
2. Cover the blender jar and then pulse for 40 to 60 seconds until smooth. Divide the drink between two glasses and then serve.

Cantaloupe Smoothie

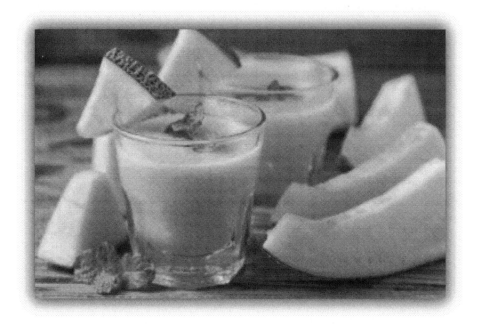

- ➢ **Preparation time:** 5 minutes
- ➢ **Servings:** 1

Ingredients:

- ½ cantaloupe, peeled, deseeded, sliced
- ¼ cup Dr. Sebi Herbal Tea
- ½ of burro banana, peeled
- ½ cup soft-jelly coconut water

Directions:

1. Plug in a high-speed food processor or blender and add all the ingredients to its jar.
2. Cover the blender jar and then pulse for 40 to 60 seconds until smooth.
3. Divide the drink between two glasses and then serve.

Watermelon Refresher

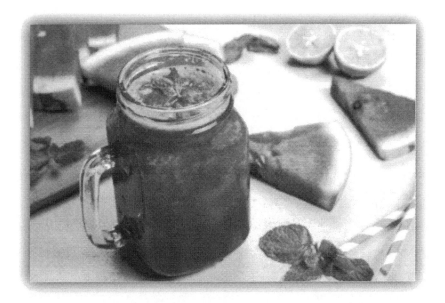

- ➢ **Preparation time:** 5 minutes
- ➢ **Servings:** 2

Ingredients:

- ½ watermelon, peeled, deseeded, cubed
- 1 tablespoon date sugar (Optional)
- ½ of key lime, juiced, zest

Directions:

1. Place watermelon pieces in a high-speed food processor or blender, add lime zest and juice, add date sugar and then pulse until smooth.
2. Take two tall glasses, fill them with a watermelon mixture until two-third full, and then pour in coconut water.
3. Stir until mixed and then serve.

Watercress Detox Smoothie

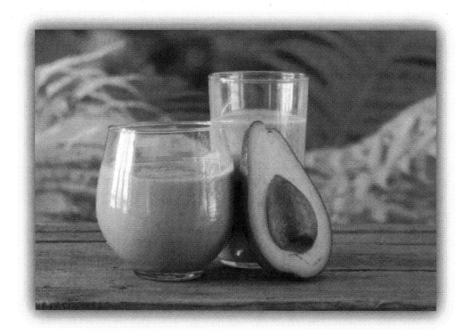

- ➤ **Preparation time:** 5 minutes
- ➤ **Servings:** 2

Ingredients:

- ½ cup watercress
- ½ of avocado, peeled, pitted
- 1 key lime, juiced
- 1 teaspoon Bromide Plus Powder (Optional)

Directions:

1. Plug in a high-speed food processor or blender and add all the ingredients to its jar.
2. Cover the blender jar and then pulse for 40 to 60 seconds until smooth.
3. Divide the drink between two glasses and then serve.

Liver Detox Smoothie Recipes

Tangy Liver Detox Smoothie

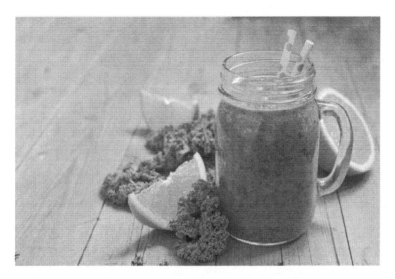

> **Preparation time:** 5 minutes
> **Servings:** 2

Ingredients:

- 2 oranges, peeled, sliced
- 1 cup shredded kalee leaves, rinsed
- 2 apples, cored, sliced
- 1 cup spring water

Directions:

1. Plug in a high-speed food processor or blender and add all the ingredients to its jar.
2. Cover the blender jar and then pulse for 40 to 60 seconds until smooth.
3. Divide the drink between two glasses and then serve.

Triple Berry Banana Smoothie

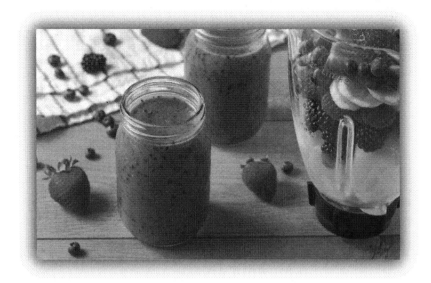

- ➢ **Preparation time:** 5 minutes
- ➢ **Servings:** 2

Ingredients:

- ½ cup strawberries
- ½ cup raspberries
- 1 burro banana, peeled
- ½ cup blueberries
- 1 cup spring water
- 2 tablespoons agave syrup (Optional)

Directions:

1. Plug in a high-speed food processor or blender and add all the ingredients to its jar.
2. Cover the blender jar and then pulse for 40 to 60 seconds until smooth.
3. Divide the drink between two glasses and then serve.

Nutty Date Papaya Smoothie

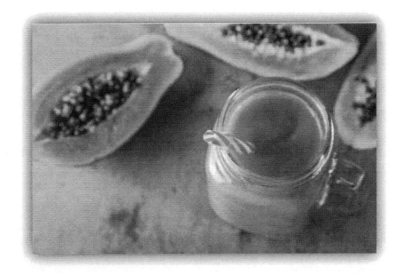

- ➢ **Preparation time:** 5 minutes
- ➢ **Servings:** 2

Ingredients:

- 1 papaya, deseeded
- 3 dates, pitted
- 1 burro banana, peeled
- ¼ of key lime, juiced
- 1 tablespoon Bromide Plus Powder (Optional)
- 1 cup spring water

Directions:

1. Plug in a high-speed food processor or blender and add all the ingredients to its jar.
2. Cover the blender jar and then pulse for 40 to 60 seconds until smooth.
3. Divide the drink between two glasses and then serve.

Dandelion & Watercress Revitalizing Smoothie

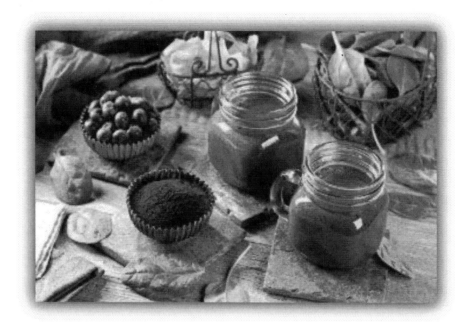

- ➢ **Preparation time:** 5 minutes
- ➢ **Servings**: 2

Ingredients:

- ¼ cup blueberries
- ½ of a large bunch of dandelion greens
- 2 baby burro bananas, peeled
- ½ cup watercress
- 3 dates, pitted
- 1 tablespoon Bromide Plus powder
- 1 cup of soft-jelly coconut water
- 2 tablespoons lime juice

Directions:

1. Plug in a high-speed food processor or blender and add all the ingredients to its jar.
2. Cover the blender jar and then pulse for 40 to 60 seconds until smooth. Divide the drink between two glasses and then serve.

BlackBerry & Burro Banana Smoothie

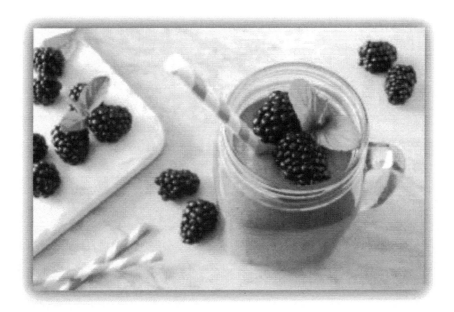

- ➤ **Preparation time:** 5 minutes
- ➤ **Servings:** 2

Ingredients:

- 1 burro banana, peeled
- ½ cup blackberries
- 2 dates, pitted
- 1 cup mango chunks
- ¼ cup walnut milk, unsweetened
- ¾ cup of coconut water

Directions:

1. Plug in a high-speed food processor or blender and add all the ingredients to its jar.
2. Cover the blender jar and then pulse for 40 to 60 seconds until smooth.
3. Divide the drink between two glasses and then serve.

Mango and Arugula Smoothie

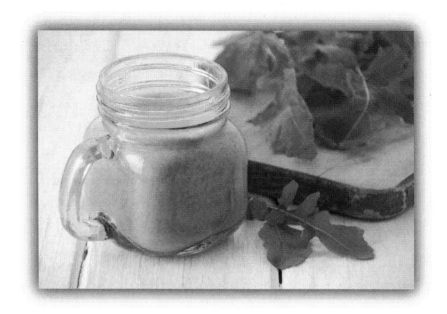

- ➢ **Preparation time:** 5 minutes
- ➢ **Servings:** 2

Ingredients:

- 1 cup mango chunks
- 2 cups arugula
- ¼ cup soft-jelly coconut, shreds
- ½ of a medium avocado, peeled, pitted
- ¾ cup of soft-jelly coconut water
- ½ of key lime, zested, juiced

Directions:

1. Plug in a high-speed food processor or blender and add all the ingredients to its jar.
2. Cover the blender jar and then pulse for 40 to 60 seconds until smooth.
3. Divide the drink between two glasses and then serve.

Refreshing Smoothie with Figs

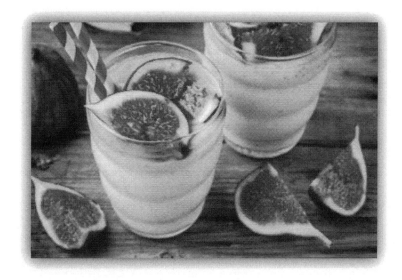

- ➢ **Preparation time:** 5 minutes
- ➢ **Servings:** 2

Ingredients:

- ½ cup of burro banana, peeled
- ½ cup figs
- 2 strawberries
- 1 cup spring water

Directions:

1. Plug in a high-speed food processor or blender and add all the ingredients to its jar.
2. Cover the blender jar and then pulse for 40 to 60 seconds until smooth.
3. Divide the drink between two glasses and then serve.

Sea moss recipes

Sea Moss Gel Recipe

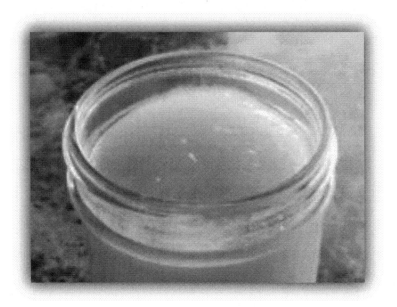

- ➢ **Preparation time:** 5 minutes
- ➢ **Servings:** 2

Ingredients:

- 1 pack organic Irish sea moss
- 1/2 cup spring water

Directions:

1. Take a pack of sea moss and cut it into chunks.
2. Wash and soak in spring water for 6 hours.
3. Drain from water.
4. Plug in a high-speed food processor or blender and add the drained sea moss and water to its jar.
5. Cover the blender jar and then pulse for 40 to 60 seconds until smooth.
6. Divide the gel between mason jars to be stored in the refrigerator or serve immediately.

Banana Mango Moss Recipe

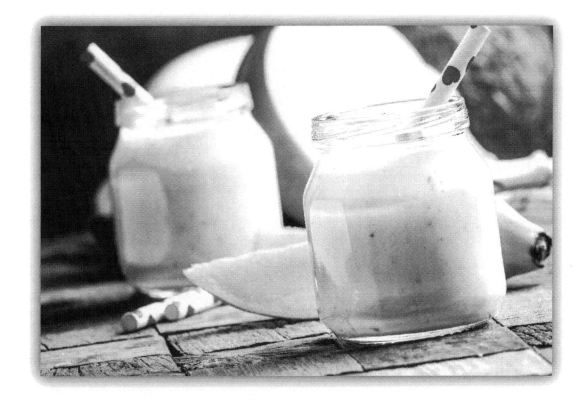

- ➢ **Preparation time:** 5 minutes
- ➢ **Servings:** 2

Ingredients:

- 1 burro banana, peeled
- ½ mango, peeled
- 1 mason jar sea moss gel
- 1 tablespoon green coconut water
- ½ cup hemp milk, homemade

Directions:

1. Take out a jar of prepared sea moss gel.
2. Plug in a high-speed food processor or blender and add all the ingredients to its jar.
3. Cover the blender jar and then pulse for 40 to 60 seconds until smooth.
4. Divide the drink between two glasses and then serve.

Creamy Sea Moss Milk Recipe

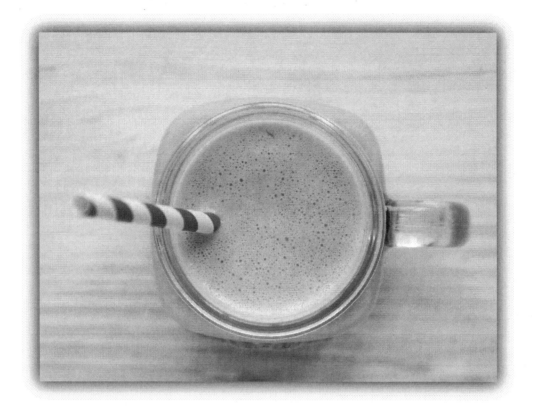

> **Preparation time:** 5 minutes
> **Servings:** 2

Ingredients:

- 1 burro banana, peeled
- ½ cup dates
- 1 mason jar sea moss gel
- ½ cup walnut milk, homemade

Directions:

1. Take out a jar of prepared sea moss gel.
2. Plug in a high-speed food processor or blender and add all the ingredients to its jar.
3. Cover the blender jar and then pulse for 40 to 60 seconds until smooth.
4. Divide the drink between two glasses and then serve.

Sea Moss Berry Shake

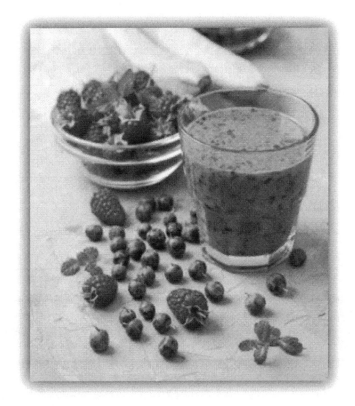

> **Preparation time:** 5 minutes
> **Servings:** 2

Ingredients:

- 1 burro banana, peeled
- ½ cup blueberries
- ½ cup raspberries
- ½ mason jar sea moss gel
- ½ cup hemp milk, homemade

Directions:

1. Take out a jar of prepared sea moss gel.
2. Plug in a high-speed food processor or blender and add all the ingredients to its jar.
3. Cover the blender jar and then pulse for 40 to 60 seconds until smooth.
4. Divide the drink between two glasses and then serve.

Sunshine Sea Moss Drink

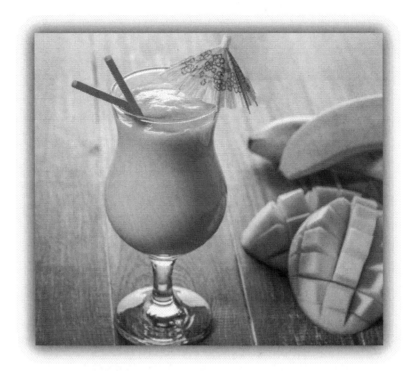

> **Preparation time:** 5 minutes
> **Servings:** 2

Ingredients:

- 1 burro banana, peeled
- ½ mango, medium, peeled and chopped
- ½ mason jar sea moss gel
- ½ cup walnut milk (optional)

Directions:

1. Take out a jar of prepared sea moss gel.
2. Plug in a high-speed food processor or blender and add all the ingredients to its jar.
3. Cover the blender jar and then pulse for 40 to 60 seconds until smooth.
4. Divide the drink between two glasses and then serve.

Smoothies for Breakfast: Boost of Energy

Avocado Blueberry Smoothie

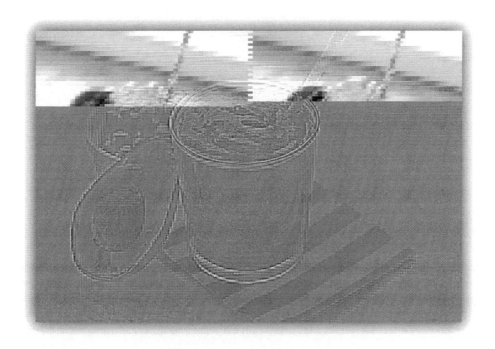

> **Preparation time:** 5 minutes
> **Servings:** 2

Ingredients:

- 1 teaspoon chia seeds
- ½ cup unsweetened coconut milk
- 1 avocado
- ½ cup blueberries

Directions:

1. Put all the fixings listed in the blender and blend until smooth and creamy.
2. Serve immediately and enjoy it.

Vegan Blueberry Smoothie

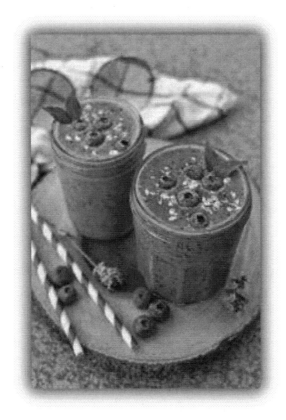

> ➢ **Preparation time**: 5 minutes
> ➢ **Servings**: 2

Ingredients:

- 2 cups blueberries
- 1 tablespoon hemp seeds
- 1 tablespoon chia seeds
- 1 tablespoon flax meal
- 1/8 teaspoon orange zest, grated
- 1 cup fresh orange juice
- 1 cup unsweetened coconut milk

Directions:

1. Toss all your ingredients into your blender, then process till smooth and creamy.
2. Serve immediately.

Berry Peach Smoothie

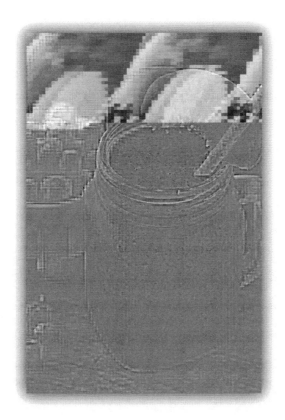

- ➢ **Preparation time**: 5 minutes
- ➢ **Servings**: 2

Ingredients:

- 1 cup of coconut water
- 1 tablespoon hemp seeds
- 1 tablespoon agave
- ½ cup strawberries
- ½ cup blueberries
- ½ cup cherries
- ½ cup peaches

Directions:

1. Toss all your berries and other fixings into your blender, then process until smooth and creamy.
2. Serve immediately.

Cantaloupe Blackberry Smoothie

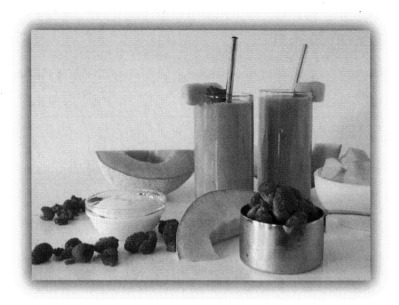

- ➢ **Preparation time**: 5 minutes
- ➢ **Servings**: 2

Ingredients:

- 1 cup coconut milk yogurt
- ½ cup raspberries
- 2 cups fresh cantaloupe
- 1 banana

Directions:

1. Toss the cantaloupe and other elements into your blender, then process till smooth.
2. Serve and enjoy.

Pineapple Kale Smoothie

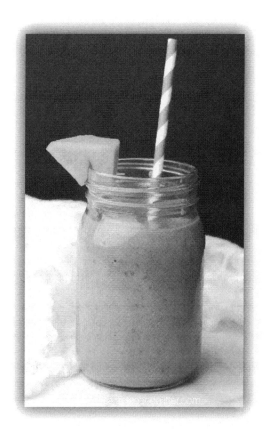

- ➢ **Preparation time**: 5 minutes
- ➢ **Servings**: 2

Ingredients:

- 8 oz. of water
- 1 orange, peeled
- 2 cups kale, chopped
- 1 banana, peeled
- 1 cup pineapple, chopped
- ½ zucchini, chopped

Directions:

1. Toss all your ingredients into your blender, then process until smooth and creamy.
2. Serve immediately.

Mix Berry Cantaloupe Smoothie

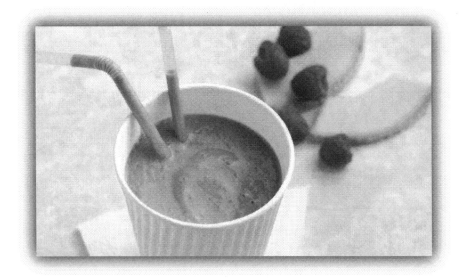

> **Preparation time**: 5 minutes
> **Servings**: 2

Ingredients:

- 1 cup alkaline water
- 2 fresh Seville orange juices
- ¼ cup fresh mint leaves
- 1 ½ cups mixed berries
- 2 cups cantaloupe

Directions:

1. Toss all your ingredients into your blender, then process until smooth.
2. Serve immediately.

Avocado Kale Smoothie

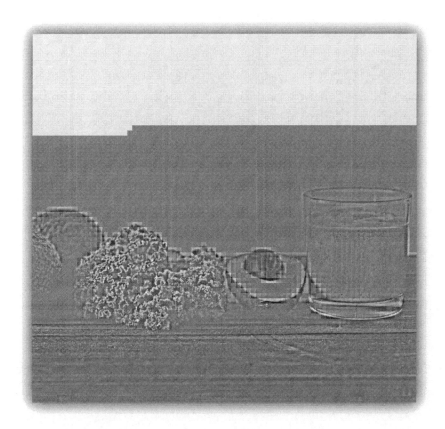

- ➢ **Preparation time**: 5 minutes
- ➢ **Servings**: 2

Ingredients:

- 1 cup of water
- ½ Seville lemon juice
- 1 avocado
- 1 cucumber, peeled
- 1 cup kale
- 1 cup of ice cubes

Directions:

1. Toss all your ingredients into your blender, then process till smooth and creamy. Serve.

Smoothies for the Brain: Improve the Connections

The Wisest Watermelon Glass

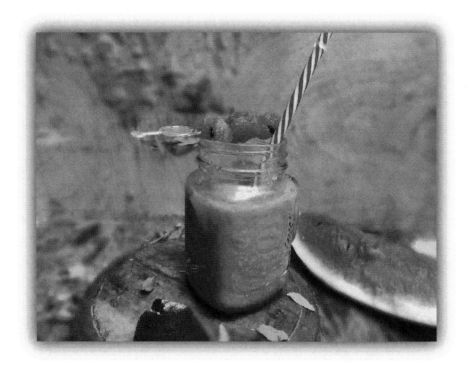

- ➤ **Preparation time:** 5 minutes
- ➤ **Servings:** 2

Ingredients:

- 1 tablespoon chia seeds
- 1 cup plain coconut yogurt
- 1 cup frozen strawberries
- 1 cup coconut milk, unsweetened
- 1 cup watermelon, chopped

Directions:

1. Add the vegetables/fruits.
2. Blend until smooth.
3. Add a few ice cubes and serve the smoothie.
4. Enjoy!

Cheery Charlie Checker

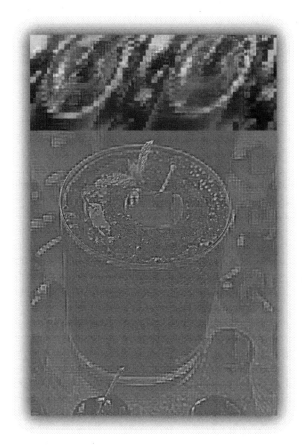

> **Preparation time:** 5 minutes
> **Servings:** 2

Ingredients:

- 1 cup coconut milk
- 1 cup frozen blueberries
- 1 fresh banana
- ¾ cup plain low-fat Greek yogurt
- ½ cup frozen cherries
- ½ cup frozen strawberries
- 1 tablespoon chia seeds

Directions:

1. Add all the ingredients in the mixer.
2. Blend until smooth.

3. Add the vegetables/fruits.
4. Blend until smooth.
5. Add a few ice cubes and serve the smoothie.
6. Enjoy!

The Pom Drink

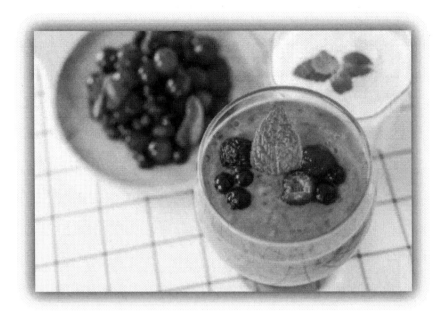

> **Preparation time:** 5 minutes
> **Servings:** 2

Ingredients:

- 1 cup plain coconut yogurt
- 1 tbsp. baby spinach
- 1 cup frozen raspberries
- 1 cup frozen blackberries
- 1 cup unsweetened vanilla coconut milk

Directions:

1. Add all the ingredients except vegetables/fruits first.
2. Blend until smooth.
3. Add the vegetables/fruits.
4. Blend until smooth.
5. Add a few ice cubes and serve the smoothie.
6. Enjoy!

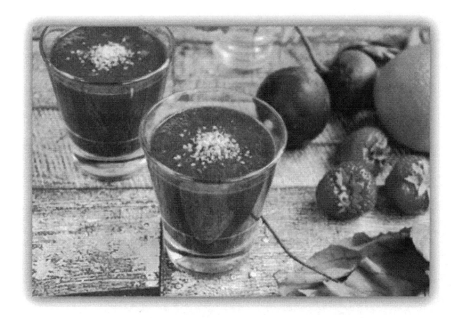

- ➢ **Preparation time:** 5 minutes
- ➢ **Servings:** 2

Ingredients:

- 1 tablespoon hemp seeds
- ¼ cup pomegranate arils
- 1 cup plain low-fat Greek yogurt
- 1 cup frozen tropical fruit mix
- 1 cup frozen strawberries
- 1 cup unsweetened vanilla almond milk

Directions:

1. Add all the ingredients in the mixer.
2. Blend until smooth.
3. Add a few ice cubes and serve the smoothie.
4. Enjoy!

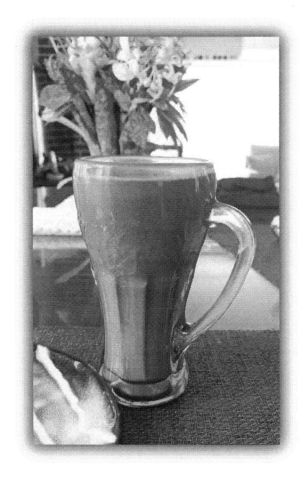

- ➤ **Preparation time:** 5 minutes
- ➤ **Servings:** 2

Ingredients:

- 1 tablespoon almond butter
- 1 tablespoon chia seeds
- 4 ice cubes
- ¾ cup plain low-fat Greek yogurt
- ½ cup diced beet
- 1 cup unsweetened almond milk
- 2 fresh bananas

Directions:

1. Add all the ingredients except vegetables/fruits first.

2. Blend until smooth.
3. Add the vegetables/fruits.
4. Blend until smooth.
5. Add a few ice cubes and serve the smoothie.
6. Enjoy!

Alkalinizing Smoothies: Stopping Acidosis

Apple Kale Cucumber Smoothie

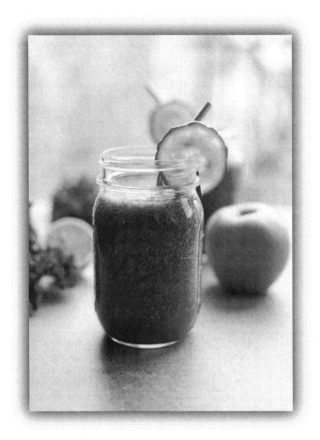

- ➢ **Preparation time**: 5 minutes
- ➢ **Servings**: 2

Ingredients:

- ¾ cup of water
- ½ green apple, diced
- ¾ cup kale
- ½ cucumber

Directions:

1. Toss all your ingredients into your blender, then process until smooth and creamy. Serve.

Refreshing Cucumber Smoothie

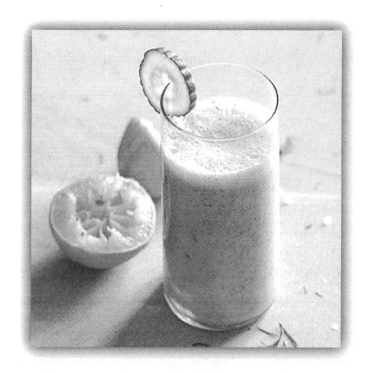

- ➢ **Preparation time**: 5 minutes
- ➢ **Servings**: 2

Ingredients:

- 2 fresh lime, peeled and halved
- 1 teaspoon lime zest, grated
- 1 cucumber, chopped
- 1 avocado, pitted and peeled
- 1 cup kale
- 1 tablespoon creamed coconut
- 1 cup of ice cubes
- 20 drops liquid stevia
- ¾ cup of coconut water

Directions:

1. Toss all your ingredients into your blender, then process until smooth and creamy. Serve.

Cauliflower Veggie Smoothie

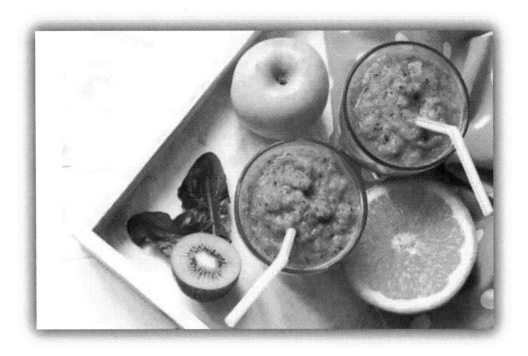

> **Preparation time**: 5 minutes
> **Servings**: 2

Ingredients:

- 1 zucchini, peeled and chopped
- 1 Seville orange, peeled
- 1 apple, diced
- 2 kiwi
- 1 cup kale
- ½ cup cauliflower

Directions:

1. Toss all your ingredients into your blender, then process until smooth and creamy. Serve.

Sweet Dream Strawberry Smoothie

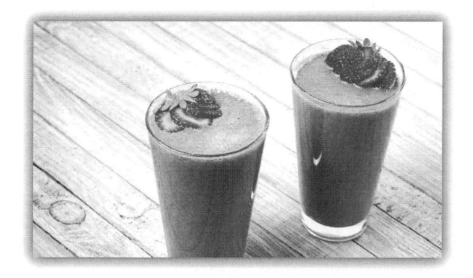

➤ **Preparation time**: 10 minutes
➤ **Servings**: 2

Ingredients:

- 5 Strawberries
- 3 dates – pits eliminated
- 2 burro bananas or small bananas
- Springwater to make 32 oz. of smoothie

Directions:

1. Peel off the skin of the bananas.
2. Wash the dates and strawberries. Add bananas, dates, and strawberries to a blender jar.
3. Add a few water and mix. Continue adding water until the mixture becomes smooth.

Alkaline Green Ginger and Banana Cleansing Smoothie

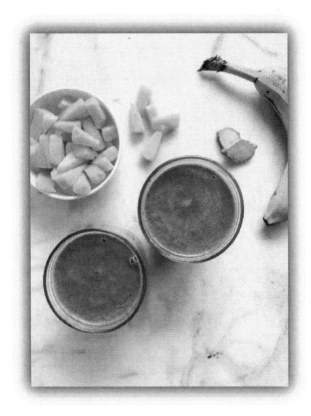

- ➢ **Preparation time**: 5 minutes
- ➢ **Servings**: 2

Ingredients:

- 1 handful of kale
- 1 banana, frozen
- 2 cups of hemp seed milk
- 1 inch of ginger, finely minced
- 1/2 cup of chopped strawberries, frozen
- 1 tablespoon of agave or your preferred sweetener

Directions:

1. Put all the ingredients in a blender and mix at high speed. Allow it to blend evenly.
2. Pour into two large glasses and serve. Enjoy!

Mixed Ananas Detox Smoothie

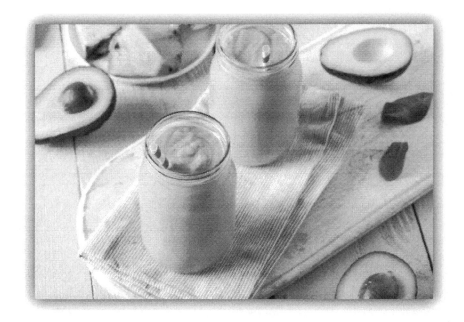

> **Preparation time**: 10 minutes
> **Servings**: 2

Ingredients:

- 1 cup of veggies (amaranth, dandelion, lettuce, or watercress)
- ½ half avocado
- 1 cup of tender-jelly coconut water
- 1 cup ananas, diced
- 1 key lime juice
- 1 tablespoon of bromide plus powder (optional)

Directions:

1. Peel and cut the Seville orange in chunks. Mix all the ingredients collectively in a high-speed blender until done.

Green Smoothie Energy: A Plenty of Chlorophyll

Post Workout Smoothie

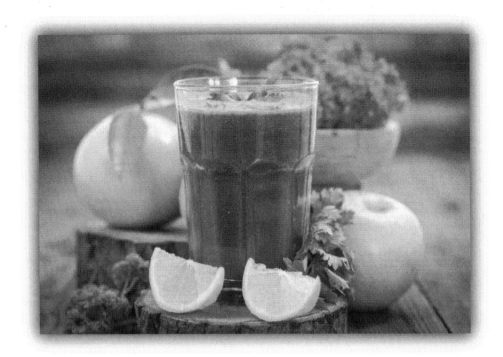

> ➤ **Preparation time:** 15 minutes
> ➤ **Servings:** 2

Ingredients:

- 1 cup dandelion greens
- ½ piece of lemon
- 1 cup celery
- 1 cup kale
- 1 piece of apple

Directions:

1. Remove the seeds from the lemon and peel it correctly.
2. Place all the ingredients in your blender.
3. Blend it for around 2 minutes.
4. Serve with a lemon slice.

Kale-cum Smoothie

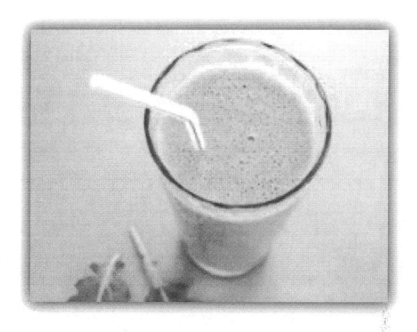

- ➤ **Preparation time:** 5 minutes
- ➤ **Servings:** 12

Ingredients:

- 1 piece apple
- 1 piece carrot
- 2 handful kale
- 1 cup pepper
- ½ cup cilantro
- 1/2 cup collard greens

Directions:

1. Cut the vegetables and fruits into cubes to fit in the binder.
2. Blend it for around 3 minutes.
3. Serve with some ice cubes.

Sprint and energy smoothie

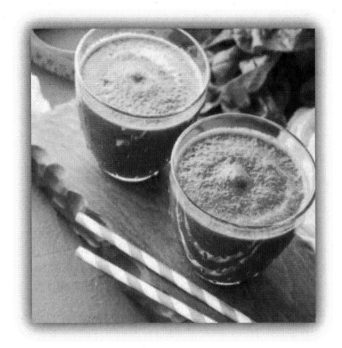

> **Preparation time:** 5 minutes
> **Servings:** 2

Ingredients:

- ½ cup blackberries
- 1 cup broccoli florets
- 1 cup spinach
- 1 green apple
- 1 teaspoon grated ginger
- - 1 cup alkaline water.

Directions:

1. Blend everything for a couple of minutes.
2. Add water if too thick.

Green Orange Smoothie

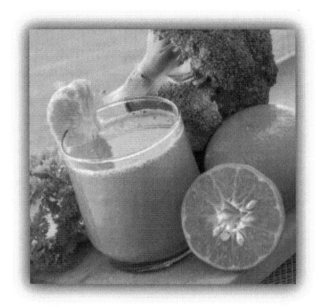

> **Preparation time:** 5 minutes
> **Servings:** 2

Ingredients:

- 2 big oranges
- ½ cup of broccoli
- 1 kiwi
- Alkaline water to taste

Directions:

1. Blend everything for a couple of minutes and strain.
2. Add water if too thick.

Detox of Spring Smoothie

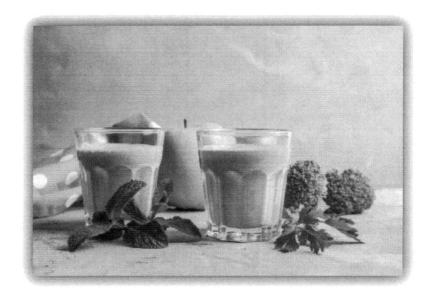

> **Preparation time:** 5 minutes
> **Servings:** 2

Ingredients:

- 1 cup of water
- ½ cup of lemon
- 1 cup kale leaves
- 1 cup dandelion green
- 1 apple, diced
- 1 pear, diced
- ½ teaspoon ginger
- ¼ teaspoon Cayenne pepper
- Honey (optional)

Directions:

1. Take all the ingredients and wash them properly.
2. Then only add everything to blender at once.
3. Blend for 3-4 minutes.
4. Take it out and use ice cubes to make it cold.

Antioxidant Smoothies: The Antiaging Therapy

Celery, Pineapple and Nopal Smoothie

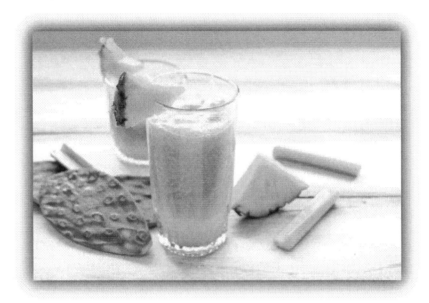

➢ **Preparation time:** 5 minutes
➢ **Servings:** 2

Ingredients:

- 1 cactus fig leaf (Nopal)
- 1 celery stalk
- 1 cup of pineapple
- 1 cup alkaline water

Directions:

1. Cut the Nopal leaf into chunks and place in blender on high speed with the celery, pineapple and water
2. Blend until smooth and homogeneous

Leafy Watermelon Cooler

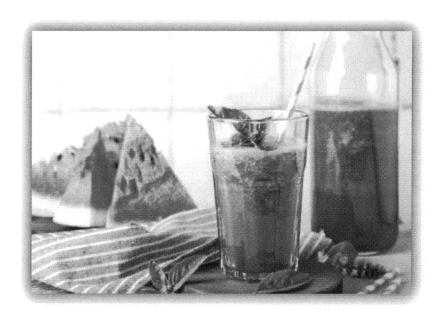

Basil has anti-bacterial and antioxidant properties that'll surely keep you healthy and young-looking while keeping you protected from most diseases. And, surprisingly, Watermelon is also full of lycopene, just like tomatoes are. This means that it can protect you against free radicals and can definitely keep you refreshed since around 75% of it is made of water!

- ➢ **Preparation time:** 5 minutes
- ➢ **Servings:** 2

Ingredients:

- 2 cups watermelon cubes, seeded
- 4 basil leaves
- ½ cup sparkling water
- 6 ice cubes

Directions:

1. Place all the ingredients in the blender or food processor and process until smooth and well-blended or for around 40 to 50 seconds.
2. Serve immediately and enjoy!

Cucumber Toxin Flush Smoothie

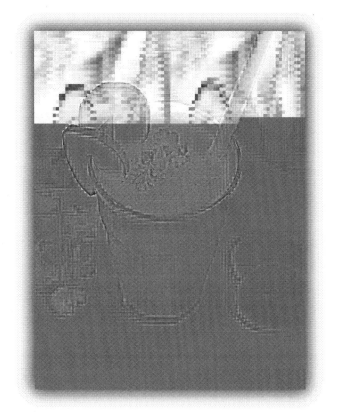

- ➤ **Preparation time:** 5 minutes
- ➤ **Servings:** 2

Ingredients:

- 1 cucumber
- 1 key lime
- 1 cup of fresh cilantro
- 1 cup alkaline water

Directions:

1. Mix all the above ingredients in a high-speed blender.
2. Juice the key lime and add it to your smoothie. Enjoy!

Cacao Flax Dandelion Shake

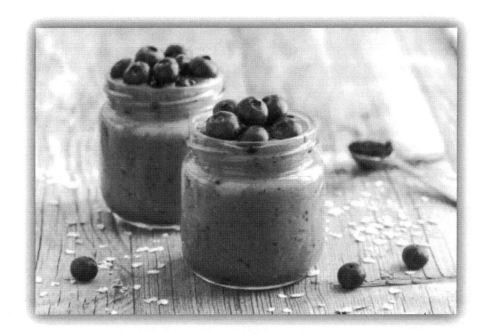

This shake is full of antioxidants that work to keep the skin healthy and beautiful. You'll also be moisturized and nourished once you try this smoothie!

➤ **Preparation time:** 5 minutes
➤ **Servings:** 2

Ingredients:

- 1 tablespoon raw cacao powder
- ½ cup organic blueberries
- 1 cup organic dandelion greens
- 1 tablespoon ground flax seeds
- 1 cup coconut water
- ½ avocado

Directions:

1. Place cacao powder, dandelion greens, blueberries, avocado, and flax seeds in the blender or food processor together with coconut water up to the max line then process until smooth and creamy or for 30 to 40 seconds.
2. Serve immediately and enjoy! Garnish with extra dandelion greens, if desired.

Blueberry Banana Smoothie

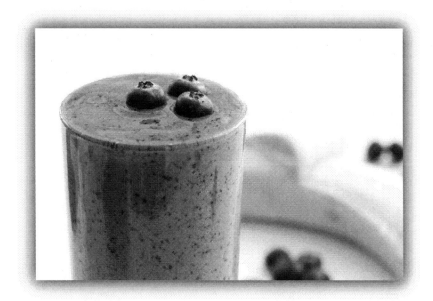

Aside from boosting metabolic levels, this smoothie works as an awesome anti-oxidant that will keep you looking healthy and radiant in no time!

- ➤ **Preparation time:** 5 minutes
- ➤ **Servings:** 2

Ingredients:

- 3 tablespoons water
- 2 teaspoons honey
- 1 green tea bag
- ½ medium banana
- ½ cups frozen blueberries
- ½ cup coconut milk

Directions:

1. Brew green tea first then add honey and stir until honey is dissolved.
2. Pour brewed green tea together with banana, blueberries, coconut milk, and water in the blender or food processor and process for around 30 to 40 seconds or until well-blended.
3. Serve topped with extra frozen blueberries, if desired. Enjoy!

Pear Broccoli Pineapple Cooler

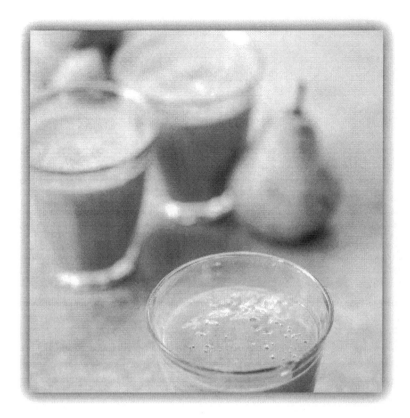

This smoothie is a great way to boost your immunity and make sure that you are protected against most diseases. It's also quite refreshing, especially on a hot summer day!

> ➢ **Preparation time:** 5 minutes
> ➢ **Servings:** 2

Ingredients:

- ½ cup pineapple chunks
- ½ cup broccoli, chopped
- Water
- 1 pear, chopped

Directions:

1. Combine pear, broccoli, and pineapple chunks in a tall glass then place in the blender or food processor together with water up to the max line.
2. Process until smooth and well-blended or for around 20 to 30 seconds.
3. Serve and enjoy!

Detox and Cleansing Smoothies: A Deep Regeneration

Green Protein Smoothie

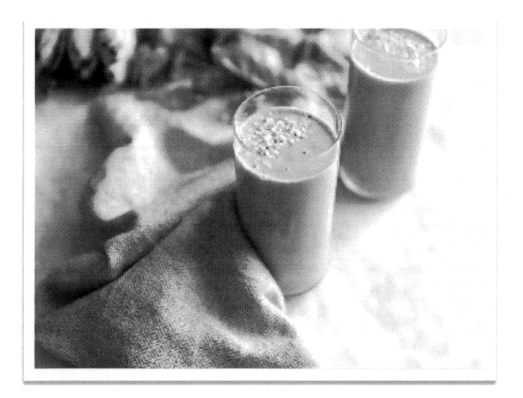

- ➤ **Preparation time:** 10 minutes
- ➤ **Servings:** 2

Ingredients:

- 1 cup unsweetened almond milk
- 2 tablespoons almond butter
- 2 bananas
- 4 cups mixed greens

Directions:

1. Add everything to a blender.
2. Blend it all into a smooth mixture.
3. Refrigerate for 2 hours or as desired.
4. Serve fresh.

Glowing Green Smoothie

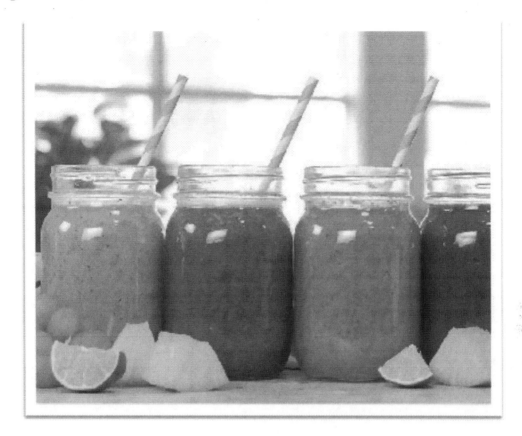

> **Preparation time:** 10 minutes
> **Servings:** 2

Ingredients:

- 2 kiwis
- 2 bananas
- ½ cup pineapple
- 4 celery stalks
- 2 cups spinach
- 2 cups alkaline water

Directions:

1. Add everything to a blender.
2. Blend it all into a smooth mixture.
3. Refrigerate for 2 hours or as desired.
4. Serve fresh.

Apple Berry Smoothie

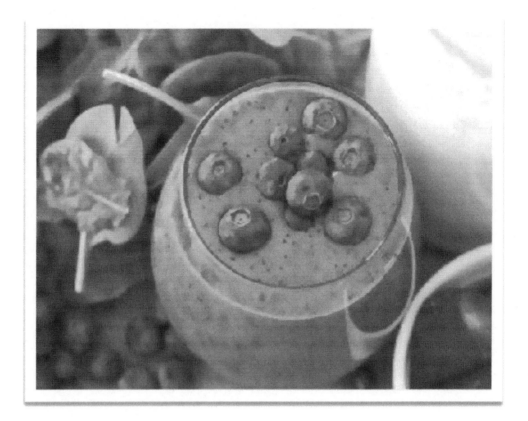

- ➢ **Preparation time:** 10 minutes
- ➢ **Servings**: 2

Ingredients:

- 2 cups mixed berries
- 2 large apples
- 4 cups spinach
- 2 cups water
-

Directions:

1. Add everything to a blender.
2. Blend it all into a smooth mixture.
3. Refrigerate for 2 hours or as desired.
4. Serve fresh.

Pineapple Banana Smoothie

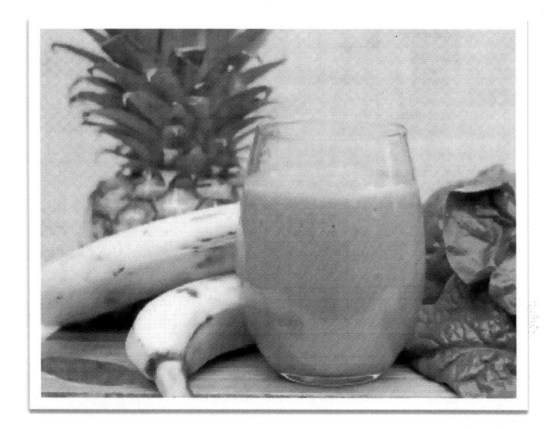

➢ **Preparation time:** 10 minutes
➢ **Servings:** 2

Ingredients:

- 2 cups pineapple
- 2 bananas
- 2 apples
- 2 cups spinach
- 2 cups water

Directions:

1. Add everything to a blender.
2. Blend it all into a smooth mixture.
3. Refrigerate for 2 hours or as desired.
4. Serve fresh.

Kale Celery Smoothie

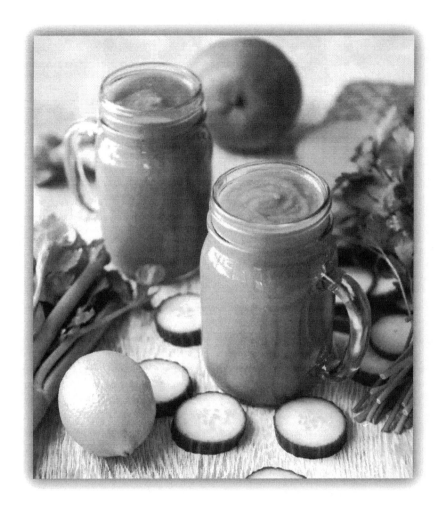

- ➢ **Preparation time:** 10 minutes
- ➢ **Servings:** 2

Ingredients:

- - 2 cups of almond milk, unsweetened
- - ½ cup of ice
- - 1 cucumber, chopped and seeded
- - 2 stalks of celery, diced
- - 1 red apple, diced
- - 1 tablespoon ground flax seeds
- - 2 teaspoons of honey
- - the juice of one lemon

Directions:

1. Add all the ingredients to a blender with ice cubes.
2. Blend well until smooth.
3. Refrigerate for 2 to 3 hours.
4. Serve.

Super Green Smoothies' Fruit-Free: The Power of Plants

Leafy Green Super Food Immune Booster

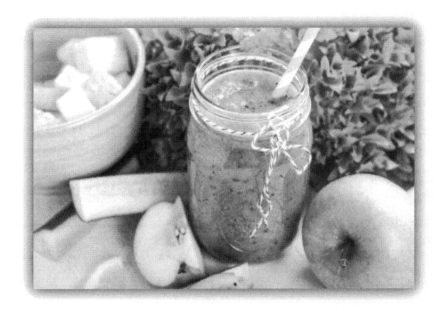

- ➤ **Preparation time:** 10 minutes
- ➤ **Servings:** 2

Ingredients:

- 6 curly salad leaves
- 1 cup diced pineapple
- 1 cucumber
- 4 stalks of celery
- 2 green apples
- 2 kiwis
- 1 teaspoon chopped ginger root

Directions:

1. Add all the ingredients to a blender with ice cubes.
2. Blend well until smooth.
3. Refrigerate for 2 to 3 hours. Serve.

Red Kale Shake

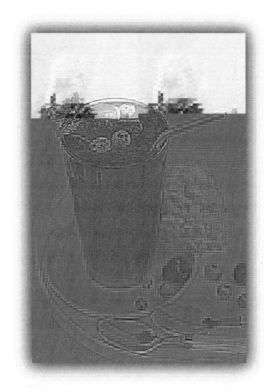

> ➤ **Preparation time:** 10 minutes
> ➤ **Servings:** 2

Ingredients:

- 1 chopped beet
- 1 cup of berries
- 2 leaves of green cabbage
- 2 kiwis
- 1 cup of coconut water
- Mint leaves for decoration

Directions:

1. Add everything to a blender.
2. Blend it all until smooth.
3. Refrigerate for 2 hours or to taste.
4. Serve chilled in two large glasses and garnish with mint leaves.

Nut Smoothie

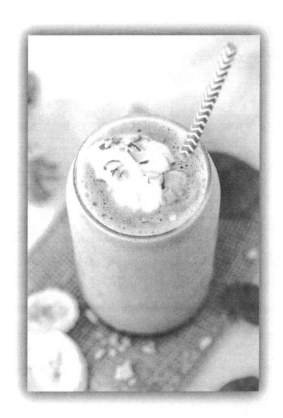

> **Preparation time:** 5 minutes
> **Servings:** 2

Ingredients:

- 3/4 cup of spinach
- 1/2 cup of carrots (shredded)
- 1 cup of almond milk
- 1/4 cup of bananas (chunked)
- 1/2 pear (no core, chopped)
- 2 tablespoons of walnuts (chopped)
- 2 tablespoons of almonds (chopped)
- 1 tablespoon of yogurt (Greek)
- 1 1/2 teaspoons of honey
- 1/4 teaspoon of cinnamon (ground)

Directions:

1. In a blender, mix all ingredients until smooth.
2. Pour the drink into a glass and enjoy.

Creamy Papaya Smoothie

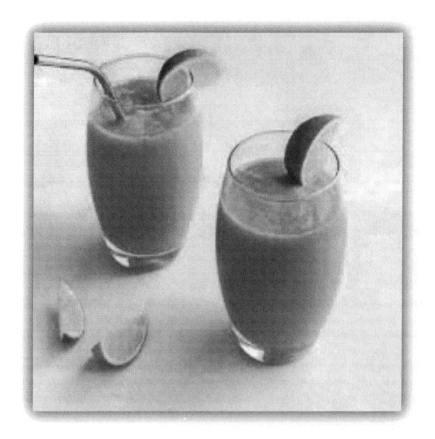

> **Preparation time:** 5 minutes
> **Servings:** 2

Ingredients:

- 1/3 cup papaya (peeled, seeded, chunked)
- 1/3 cup of coconut milk
- 1/3 cup of ice
- 2 teaspoons honey
- 2 tbsp. of almond cream

Directions:

1. In a blender, combine all ingredients
2. Blend until smooth.
3. Serve the smoothie in large glasses with lime or lemon slices, and enjoy.

Strawberry Mud Smoothie

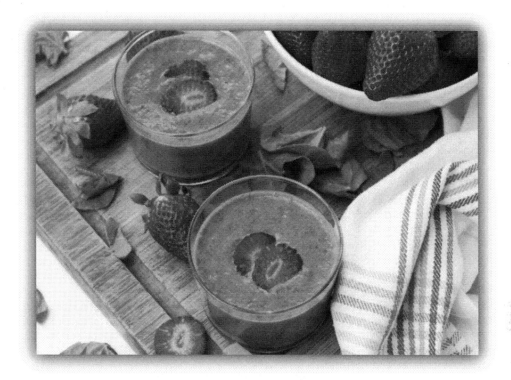

- ➢ **Preparation time:** 5 minutes
- ➢ **Servings:** 2

Ingredients:

- 1/2 cup of spinach (frozen)
- 1/2 cup of strawberries (frozen)
- 1/4 cup of banana (chunked)
- 2 tablespoons of ice
- 1 1/2 teaspoon of honey

Directions:

1. In a blender add all the 1/2 cup of spinach (frozen), 1/2 cup of strawberries (frozen), 1/4 cup of banana (chunked), 2 tablespoons of ice, and 1 1/2 teaspoon of honey and blend until smooth. Pour in a glass and enjoy.

Zucchini Orange Smoothie

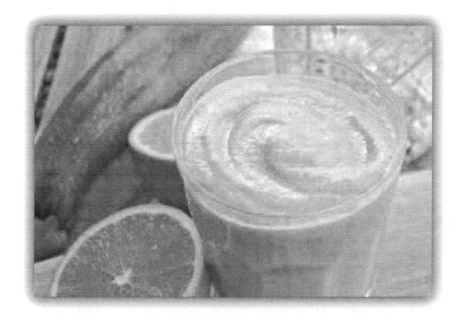

- ➤ **Preparation time:** 5 minutes
- ➤ **Servings:** 2

Ingredients:

- 1/2 of a zucchini (cubed)
- 3 ice cubes
- 1/2 cup of orange juice
- 1 tablespoon of honey
- 1/4 teaspoon of vanilla extract

Directions:

1. In a blender, add 1/2 of a zucchini (cubed), 3 ice cubes, 1/2 cup orange juice, 1 tablespoon of honey, and 1/4 teaspoon of vanilla extract and blend until smooth. Pour in a glass and enjoy.

Silly Sweet Zucchini Smoothie

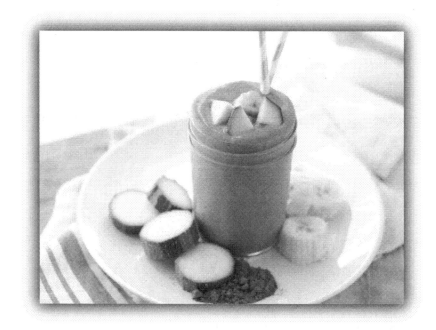

➢ **Preparation time:** 5 minutes
➢ **Servings:** 2

Ingredients:

- ¼ cup of zucchini (grated and frozen)
- ½ banana (chunked)
- ½ cup of coconut cream
- ½ tablespoon of cocoa powder
- 1 tablespoon of macadamia nuts (finely chopped)
- 1 pinch of vanilla essence

Directions:

1. Pour all ingredients into a blender.
2. Blend until smooth.
3. Pour into a glass and enjoy the drink.

Low-Sugar Smoothies: Keep a Low Insulin Level

Low-Sugar Lime & Basil Green Juice

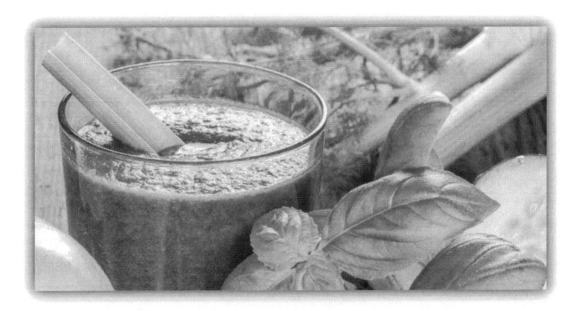

- ➤ **Preparation time:** 5 minutes
- ➤ **Servings:** 1

Ingredients:

- 70 ml chilled apple juice
- 70 ml chilled celery juice
- 50 g baby spinach
- 20 g basil leaves
- 1 cucumber, chopped
- 1 lime, zested and juiced

Directions:

1. Pour the apple juice into a large jug and then add the spinach, basil, cucumber, lime, and 100 ml chilled water.
2. Blitz well with a hand blender until smooth. Pour into a glass and drink straight away.

Apple Blueberry Smoothie

> ➤ **Preparation time**: 10 minutes
> ➤ **Servings**: 2

Ingredients:

- ½ apple
- 1 date
- ½ cup of blueberries
- 1 tablespoon of hemp seeds
- 1 tablespoon of sesame seeds
- 2 cups of sparkling soft-jelly coconut water

Directions:

1. Mix all the fixings in a high-speed blender and enjoy!
- Protein: 6.7 g

Detox Berry Smoothie

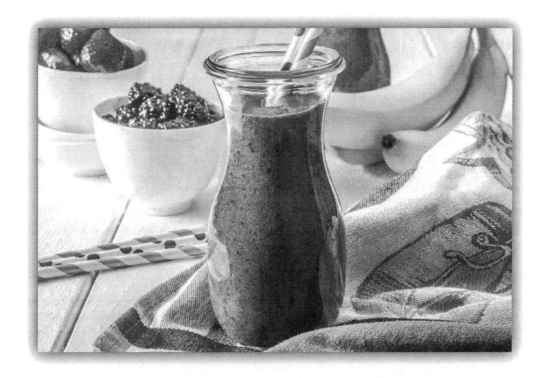

- ➢ **Preparation time**: 10 minutes
- ➢ **Servings**: 2

Ingredients:

- Springwater
- 1/4 avocado, pitted
- 1 medium burro banana
- 1 Seville orange
- 2 cups of fresh lettuce
- 1 tablespoon of hemp seeds
- 1 cup of berries (blueberries or an aggregate of blueberries, strawberries, and raspberries)

Directions:

1. Add the spring water to your blender. Put the fruits and veggies right inside the blender.
2. Blend all ingredients till smooth. Serve.

Papaya Detox Smoothie

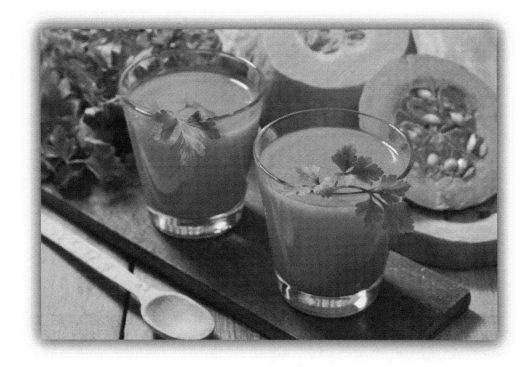

> ➤ **Preparation time:** 10 minutes
> ➤ **Servings:** 2

Ingredients:

- 1 cup butternut squash
- 1 tablespoon of chopped ginger root
- 1 cup alkaline water
- a few sprigs of parsley

Directions:

1. Chop the papaya into square portions and scoop out a tablespoon of clean and raw papaya seeds.
- Pour smoothie into two glasses, sprinkle with parsley leaves, and serve.

Apple and Amaranth Detoxifying Smoothie

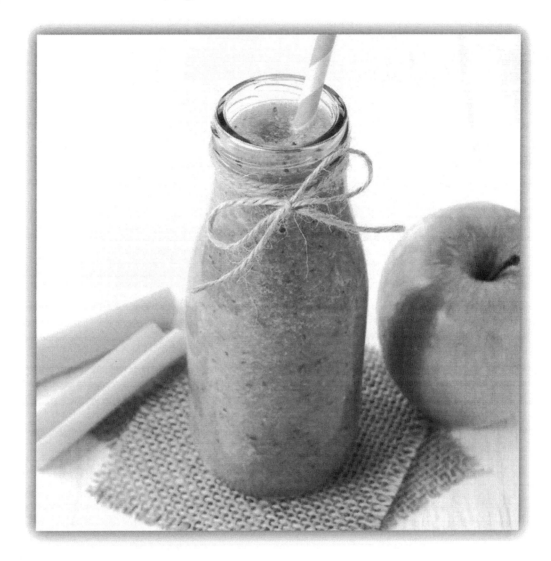

> **Preparation time:** 10 minutes
> **Servings:** 2

Ingredients:

- ½ avocado
- 1 key lime juice
- 2 apples, chopped
- 2 cups of water
- 2 cups of Amaranth vegie

Directions:

1. Put all the ingredients collectively in a blender.
2. Blend all the ingredients evenly.
3. Enjoy this delicious smoothie.

Avocado Mixed Smoothie

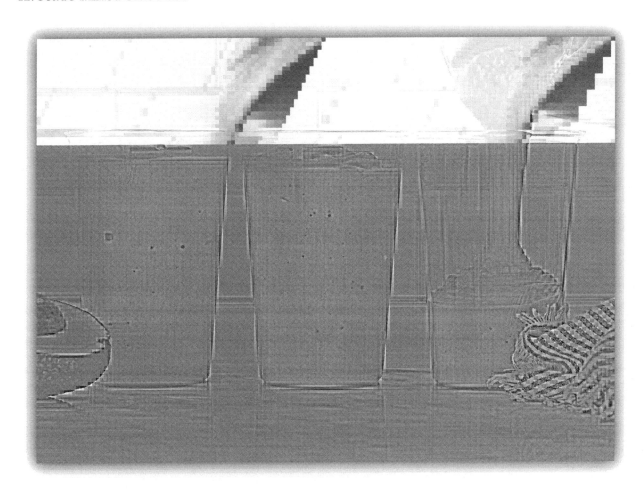

> **Preparation time:** 10 minutes
> **Servings:** 3

Ingredients:

- 1 cup alkaline water
- 1 pear, chopped
- 1 avocado, pitted
- 1/4 cup coconut flakes
- Juice of half a lemon

Directions:

1. Blend all components in a high-speed blender and refrigerate.

2. After one hour, pour the smoothie into three large glasses and enjoy.

Peach Berry Smoothie

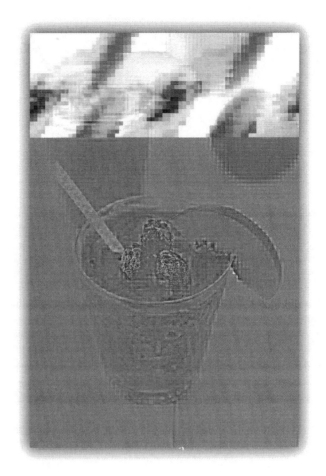

> **Preparation time:** 10 minutes
> **Servings:** 4

Ingredients:

- ½ cup of frozen peaches
- ½ cup of frozen blueberries
- ½ cup of frozen cherries
- ½ cup of frozen strawberries
- 1 tablespoon of sea moss gel
- 1 tablespoon of hemp seeds
- 1 tablespoon of coconut water
- 1 tablespoon of agave

Directions:

1. Put all the above fixings in a blender and blend for one minute.
2. If the combination is too thick, add extra coconut water and blend for another 20 secs.
3. Enjoy your peach berry smoothie!

Digestive Smoothie: Stop Stomach Bloating

Tropical Storm Glass

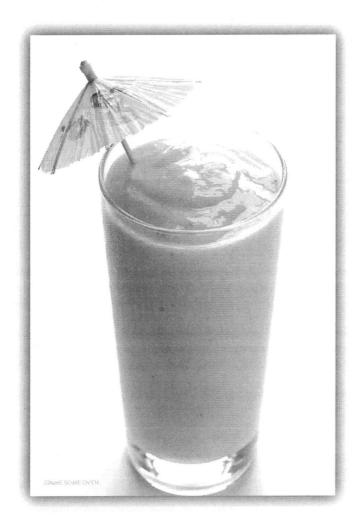

> **Preparation time:** 5 minutes
> **Servings:** 2

Ingredients:

- ½ cup of coconut yogurt
- 1 cup unsweetened coconut milk
- 1 fresh banana
- 1 cup frozen tropical fruit (mix of papaya, mango and pineapple)

Directions:

1. Add all the ingredients.
2. Blend until smooth.
3. Add a few ice cubes and serve the smoothie.
4. Enjoy!

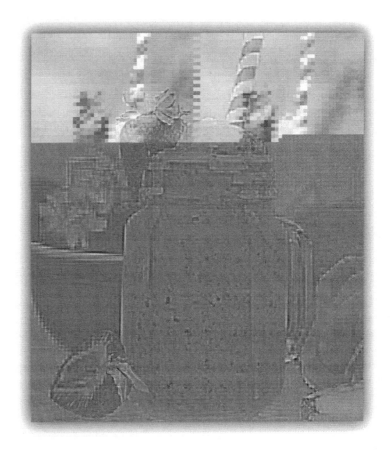

> **Preparation time:** 5 minutes
> **Servings:** 2

Ingredients:

- ½ cup water
- ¾ cup greek yogurt
- 1 cup frozen peaches
- 1 cup baby spinach
- 1 cup frozen mixed berries
- 1 cup unsweetened vanilla almond milk

Directions:

1. Add all the ingredients except vegetables/fruits first.
2. Blend until smooth.
3. Add the vegetables/fruits.

4. Blend until smooth.
5. Add a few ice cubes and serve the smoothie.
6. Enjoy!

Nutrition:

- Calories: 167
- Fat: 6 g
- Carbs: 25 g
- Protein: 8 g

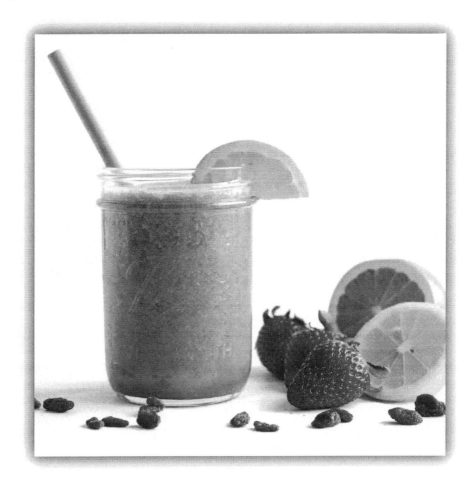

➢ **Preparation time:** 5 minutes
➢ **Servings:** 2

Ingredients:

- 1 squeezed clementine
- 1 squeezed blood orange
- ¾ cup low-fat Greek yogurt
- 1 cup of frozen strawberries
- 1 cup of Cantaloupe melon
- 1 cup unsweetened almond milk

Directions:

1. Add all the ingredients.
2. Blend until smooth.
3. Add a few ice cubes and serve the smoothie.
4. Enjoy!

A Minty Drink

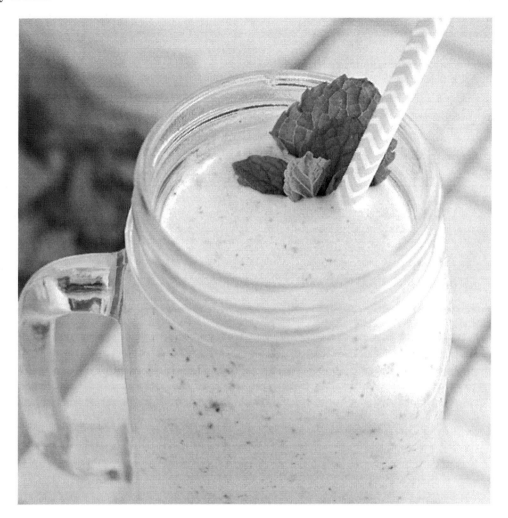

- ➢ **Preparation time:** 5 minutes
- ➢ **Servings:** 2

Ingredients:

- 1 tablespoon hemp seeds
- Fresh mint leaves
- ¾ cup plain coconut yogurt
- 1 cup frozen mango
- 1 cup frozen strawberries
- 1 cup unsweetened vanilla almond milk

Directions:

1. Add all the ingredients.
2. Blend until smooth.
3. Add a few ice cubes and serve the smoothie.
4. Enjoy your smoothie!

The Baked Apple

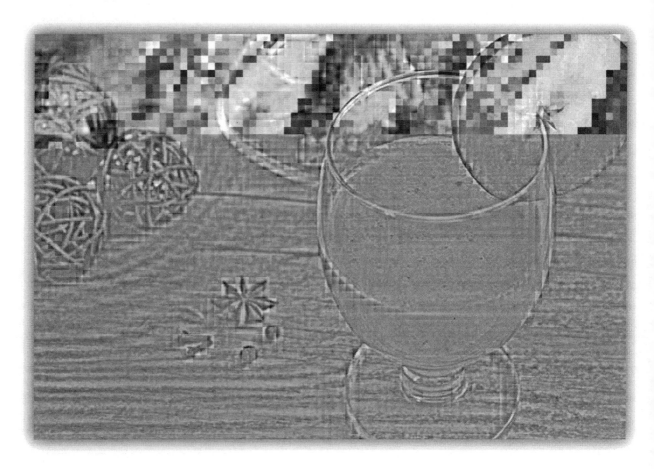

- ➤ **Preparation time:** 5 minutes
- ➤ **Servings:** 2

Ingredients:

- Dash ground cinnamon
- 1 tablespoon rolled oats
- 1 tablespoon hemp seeds
- ¾ cup Greek yogurt
- 1 cup pear chunks
- 1 cup apple chunks
- 1 cup unsweetened almond milk

Directions:

1. Add all the ingredients.
2. Blend until smooth.
3. Add a few ice cubes and serve the smoothie.
4. Enjoy!

High Energy Smoothies: For Top Performance

Great Green Garden

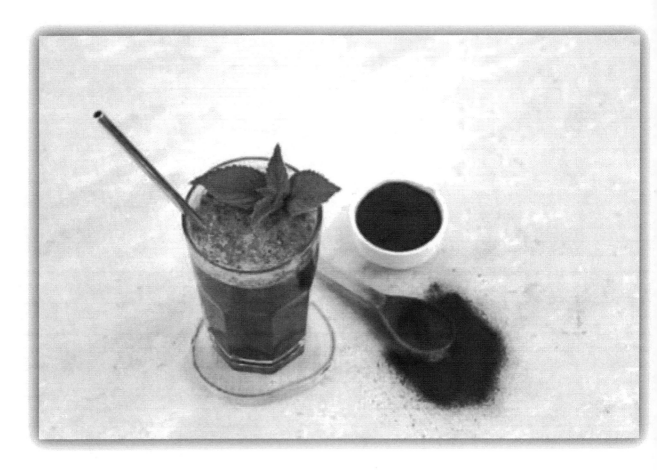

- ➢ **Preparation time:** 5 minutes
- ➢ **Servings:** 2

Ingredients:

- 1 teaspoon spirulina
- Few fresh mints leave
- ½ cup cucumber, peeled
- 1 cup unsweetened coconut milk
- 3 ice cubes

Directions:

1. Add all the ingredients.
2. Blend until smooth.

3. Add a few ice cubes and serve the smoothie.
4. Enjoy!

Spirulina Surprise

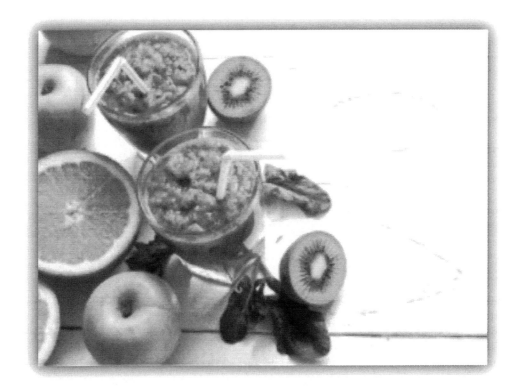

- ➤ **Preparation time:** 5 minutes
- ➤ **Servings:** 2

Ingredients:

- 1 tablespoon of spirulina
- 2 green apples, chopped
- 1 cup of spinach leaves
- 2 kiwis, chopped
- 1 orange, juiced

Directions:

1. Add all the ingredients.
2. Blend until smooth.
3. Add a few ice cubes and serve the smoothie.
4. Enjoy!

Powerful Purple Smoothie

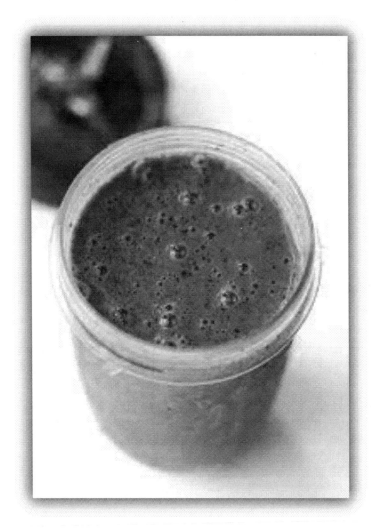

- ➤ **Preparation time:** 5 minutes
- ➤ **Servings:** 2

Ingredients:

- 1 tablespoon of powdered wheat grass
- 1 tablespoon spirulina
- 1 frozen banana, sliced
- 2 packages of frozen acaj berries
- 1 cup baby spinach

- 1 cup coconut water

Directions:

1. Add all the ingredients in the mixer
2. Blend until smooth.
3. Add a few ice cubes and serve the smoothie.
4. Enjoy!

Health Blast

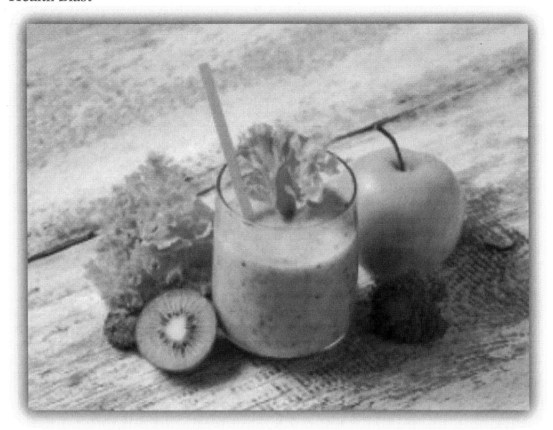

- ➤ **Preparation time:** 5 minutes
- ➤ **Servings:** 2

Ingredients:

- 1 teaspoon of bee pollen
- 2 fresh kiwis
- 2 green apples
- 1 cup chopped curly lettuce
- ½ cup broccoli florets
- 1½ cups unsweetened coconut milk drink
- 1 cup ice

Directions:

1. Add all ingredients except vegetables first.
2. Blend for 30 seconds.
3. Combine vegetables.
4. Blend until smooth.
5. Add a few ice cubes and serve the smoothie.

Weight Loss Smoothies: Ideal for for increasing Lean Mass

Slim-Jim Vanilla Latte

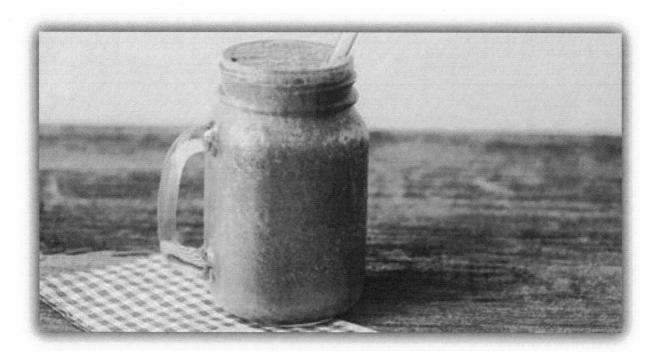

- ➢ **Preparation time:** 5 minutes
- ➢ **Servings:** 2

Ingredients:

- 2 fresh bananas
- 1 green apple
- A pinch of cinnamon powder
- 1 tablespoon chia seeds
- ½ cup unsweetened almond milk
- ½ cup of chicory coffee
- 4 ice cubes

Directions:

1. Add all the ingredients except vegetables/fruits first.
2. Blend until smooth.

3. Add the vegetables/fruits.

4. Blend until smooth.

5. Add a few ice cubes and serve the smoothie.

6. Enjoy!

Cauliflower Cold Glass

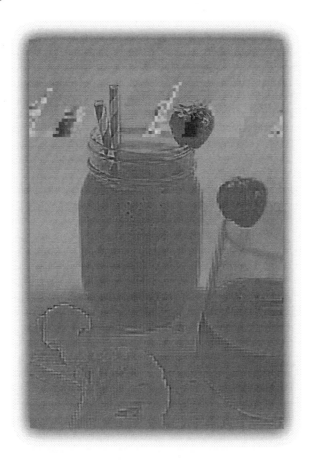

- ➢ **Preparation time:** 5 minutes
- ➢ **Servings:** 2

Ingredients:

- ½ cup grated cauliflower
- ½ cup frozen strawberries
- ½ cup frozen blueberries
- ¾ cup low-fat Greek yogurt
- 1 fresh banana
- 1 cup unsweetened coconut milk

Directions:

1. Add all the ingredients in the mixer
2. Blend until smooth.
3. Add a few ice cubes and serve the smoothie.
4. Enjoy!

Anti-aging Papaya and Goji Smoothie

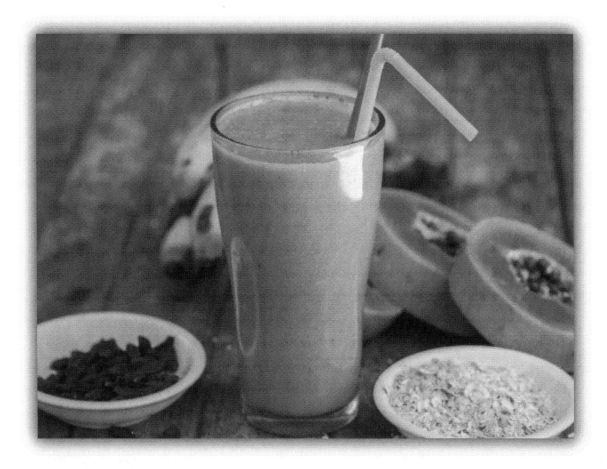

- ➢ **Preparation time:** 5 minutes
- ➢ **Servings:** 2

Ingredients:

- 1 cup chopped papaya
- 1 tablespoon goji berries
- ¾ cup low-fat Greek yogurt
- ½ frozen banana cut into chunks
- 2 tablespoons gluten-free rolled oatmeal
- 1 cup unsweetened almond milk

Directions:

1. Soak the goji berries half an hour before.
2. Place all ingredients in blender.
3. Blend.
4. Add a few ice cubes and serve the smoothie.

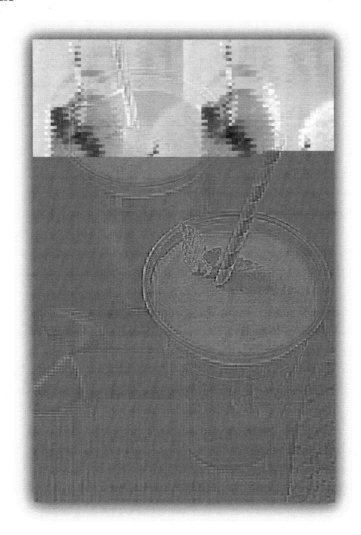

- ➤ **Preparation time:** 5 minutes
- ➤ **Servings:** 2

Ingredients:

- ½ cup fresh avocado
- ½ cup plain coconut yogurt
- 1 fresh banana
- 1 cup baby spinach
- 1 cup frozen mango
- 1 cup unsweetened coconut milk

Directions:

1. Add all ingredients except baby spinach first.
2. Blend until smooth.
3. Add spinach.
4. Blend until creamy.
5. Add a few mint leaves and serve the smoothie.

The Summer Hearty Shake

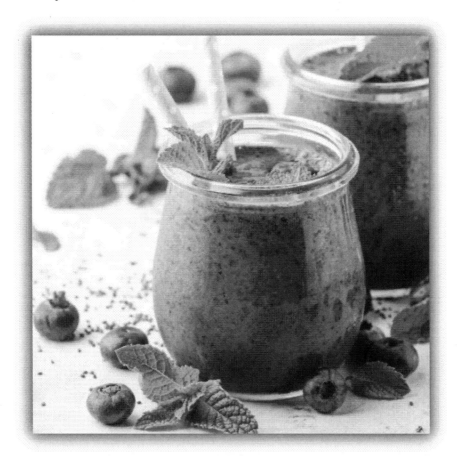

> **Preparation time:** 5 minutes
> **Servings:** 2

Ingredients:

- 1 cup frozen blackberries
- ½ cup frozen blueberries
- 1 cup coconut milk
- 1 tablespoon hemp seeds
- A pinch of cinnamon powder

Directions:

1. Combine all ingredients in blender.
2. Blend until smooth.
3. Add a few ice cubes and serve the smoothie.

Protein Smoothies: Muscle Power

Cocoa Tofu Smoothie

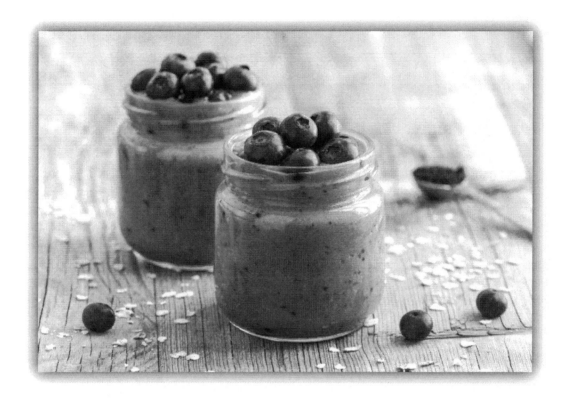

- ➤ **Preparation time:** 5 minutes
- ➤ **Servings:** 2

Ingredients:

- 1/2 cup of milk
- 1/4 cup of tofu (silken, chunked)
- 1/4 cup of banana (chunks)
- 1/3 tablespoon of honey
- 2/3 tablespoon of chocolate drink mix
- 1/8 tablespoon of wheat germ

Directions:

1. Blend all ingredients until smooth.
2. Pour into a glass and top with blueberries.
3. Can be enjoyed by the spoonful.

Banana Berry Tofu Smoothie

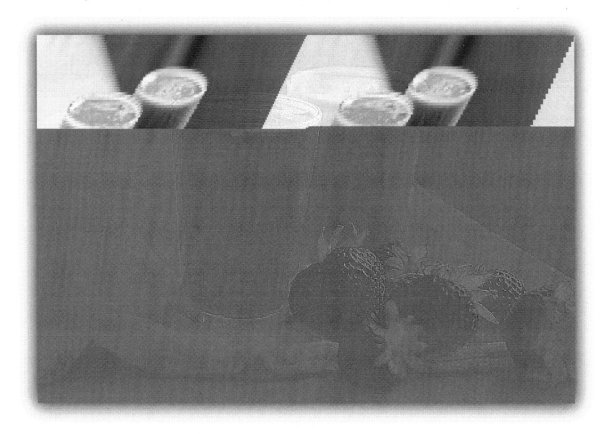

> **Preparation time:** 5 minutes
> **Servings:** 2

Ingredients:

- 1/2 cup of strawberries
- 1/3 cup blueberries
- 1 banana
- ½ cup unsweetened almond milk
- ¼ cup fermented tofu cubes
- ¼ cup blueberries
- 1 cup alkaline water

Directions:

1. Add all the ingredients in the mixer
2. Blend until smooth.
3. Add a few ice cubes and serve the smoothie.
4. Enjoy!

Apple Strawberry Banana Smoothie

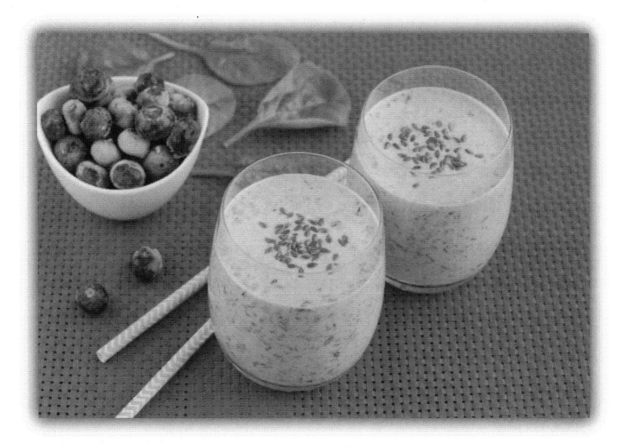

- ➢ **Preparation time:** 5 minutes
- ➢ **Servings:** 2

Ingredients:

- 1 banana
- ½ cup fresh blueberries
- 1/4 cup baby spinach
- 1 cup spring water
- 3 ice cubes
- ½ tablespoon honey
- 1 teaspoon flax seeds + seeds for decoration

Directions:

1. Pour all ingredients, except spinach, into blender and blend for about 30 seconds
2. Add the spinach leaves and ice cubes and continue blending to make a smooth mixture
3. Pour into two large glasses and cover with some linseed.
4. Keep in the fridge at least half an hour before serving to allow the flax seeds to release their gel
5. Remove from the fridge and enjoy

Apple Peach Banana Smoothie

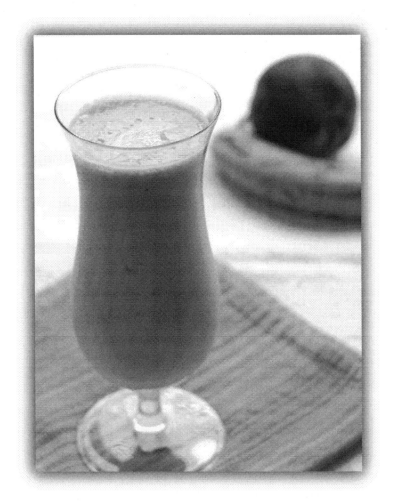

> **Preparation time:** 5 minutes
> **Servings:** 2

Ingredients:

- ½ cup peaches (sliced)
- ¼ cup apple juice
- ¼ cup cashew cream cheese
- ½ cup frozen banana (sliced)
- 4 ice cubes
- 1/2 tablespoon honey
- 2 slices of peach

Directions:

1. Blend all ingredients except peach slice until smooth.
2. Pour into a glass, garnish with a peach slice and enjoy the drink.

Smoothies for Healthy Skin and Hair: More Freshness and Hydration

Evergreen Morning Dew

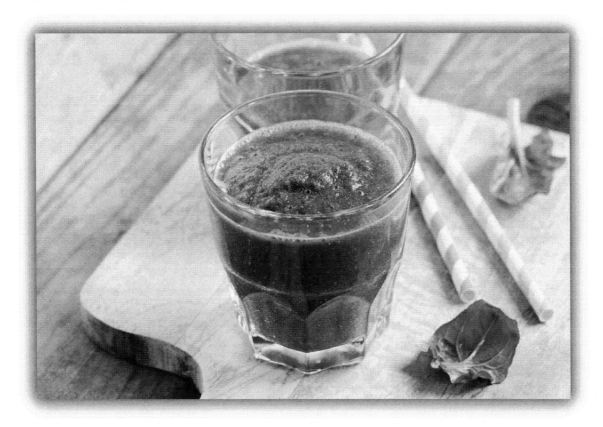

- ➢ **Preparation time:** 5 minutes
- ➢ **Servings:** 2

Ingredients:

- 1 cup cabbage, cut into small pieces
- ½ cup broccoli florets
- 1 kiwi
- ½ cup ice
- 1 tablespoon collagen protein powder
- Pinch of cayenne
- 1/2 lemon, juiced
- 1 cup of water

Directions:

1. Add all ingredients except spinach leaves.
2. Blend for 30 seconds.
3. Add spinach leaves.
4. Blend until smooth.
5. Add a few ice cubes and serve the smoothie.

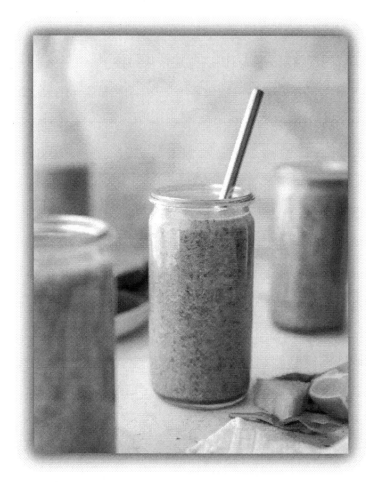

> **Preparation time:** 5 minutes
> **Servings:** 2

Ingredients:

- ½ cup frozen ananas
- ½ cup seeded cucumber, diced
- 1 cup collard greens, chopped
- 3 stalks celery, chopped
- ½ teaspoon fresh ginger, peeled and minced
- ¼ cup fresh flat-leaf parsley, chopped
- 1 scoop collagen protein powder

- 1 tablespoon freshly squeezed lemon juice
- 1 tablespoon freshly squeezed lime juice
- ½ cup water

Directions:

1. Add all the ingredients in the mixer
2. Blend until smooth.
3. Add a few ice cubes and serve the smoothie.
4. Enjoy!

Exotic Reishi Pear

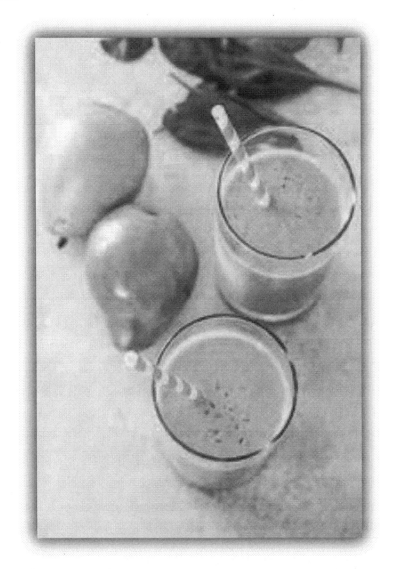

> **Preparation time:** 10 minutes
> **Servings:** 2

Ingredients:

- 1 cup baby spinach
- 1 pear, roughly chopped
- ¼ cup raw cashews
- 1 teaspoon reishi mushroom powder
- 1 cup unsweetened cashew milk

- ½ cup ice

Directions:

1. Add all ingredients except spinach leaves.
2. Blend for 30 seconds.
3. Add spinach leaves.
4. Blend until smooth.
5. Add a few ice cubes and serve the smoothie.
6. Enjoy!

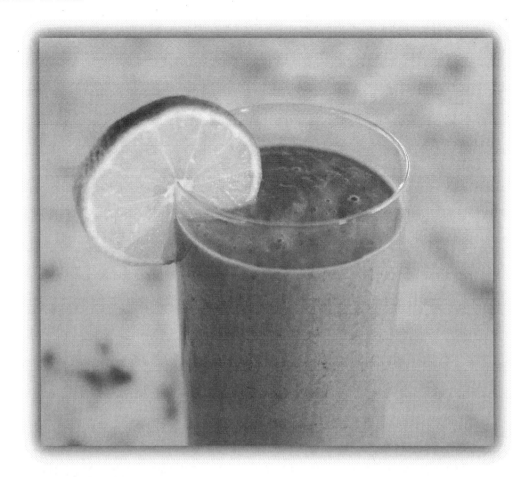

> **Preparation time:** 5 minutes
> **Servings:** 2

Ingredients:

- 5 large leaves of romaine lettuce
- ½ cucumber, diced
- 3 celery stalks, chopped
- 1 carrot, shredded
- 1 orange, peeled and segmented
- 10 drops vitamin D
- ½ cup water
- 4 ice cubes

Directions:

1.   Pour all ingredients into blender.
2.   Blend until smooth.
3.   Serve immediately in high glasses.

Vitamin smoothie for your skin

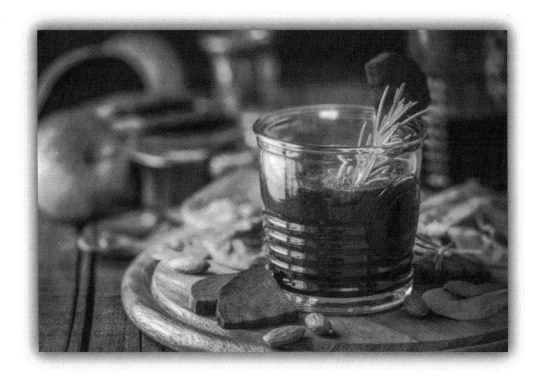

- ➤ **Preparation time:** 10 minutes
- ➤ **Servings:** 2

Ingredients:

- 1½ cups beets, chopped
- ½ grapefruit, juiced
- 1 orange, juiced
- ½ small apple, chopped
- 1 cup baby spinach
- 1 tablespoon chopped almonds
- 1 tablespoon collagen protein powder
- 1 cup rosemary infusion

Directions:

1. Pour the rosemary infusion, almonds, apples, and collagen into the blender.

2. Blend for about 30 seconds.
3. Add remaining ingredients and continue blending.
4. Add a few ice cubes and a sprig of rosemary for decoration and serve.

Herbal Tea Recipes

Liver-Kidney Cleansing Tea

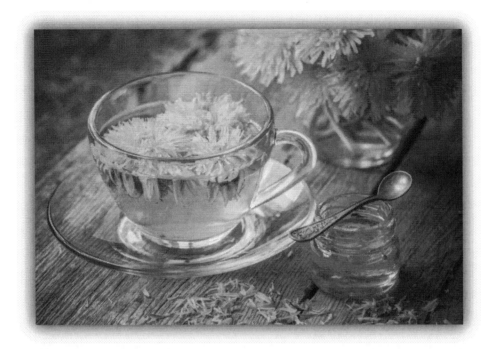

- ➢ **Preparation time:** 5 minutes
- ➢ **Cooking time:** 10 minutes
- ➢ **Servings:** 2

Ingredients:

- 1 teaspoon dandelion root powder
- 1 teaspoon burdock root powder
- 1 cup spring water

Directions:

1. Place all ingredients in a tea kettle.
2. Boil for 10 minutes and remove it from heat, cover, and leave for an additional 10 minutes.

3. Drain and serve.

Nutrition:

- Calories: 98
- Fats: 2 g
- Carbs: 3 g
- Protein: 4 g
- Fiber: 5 g

Refreshing Kidney Cleansing Tea

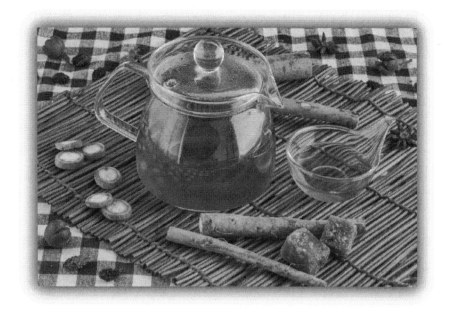

- ➢ **Preparation time:** 5 minutes
- ➢ **Cooking time:** 10 minutes
- ➢ **Servings:** 2

Ingredients:

- 1 teaspoon Prodigiosa powder.
- 1 teaspoon burdock root powder.
- 1 cup spring water.

Directions:

1. Place all ingredients in a tea kettle.
2. Boil for 10 minutes and remove it from heat, cover, and leave for an additional 10 minutes.
3. Drain and serve.

Nutrition:

- Calories: 85
- Fats: 6 g
- Carbs: 7 g
- Protein: 2 g
- Fiber: 6 g

Mucus Liver Cleansing Tea

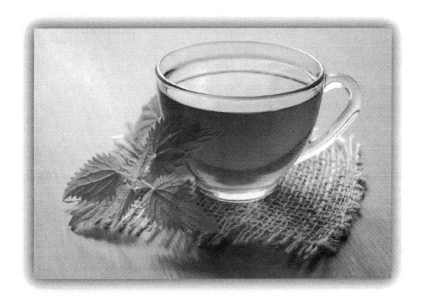

- ➤ **Preparation time:** 5 minutes
- ➤ **Cooking time:** 10 minute
- ➤ **Servings:** 1

Ingredients:

- 1 teaspoon dandelion root powder
- 1 teaspoon Prodigiosa powder
- Mint leaves
- 1 cup spring water

Directions:

1. Place all ingredients in a tea kettle.
2. Boil for 10 minutes and remove it from heat, cover, and leave for an additional 10 minutes.
3. Drain and serve.

Nutrition:

- Calories: 30
- Fat: 2.5 g
- Carbs: 0.5 g
- Protein: 1.5 g
- Fiber: 11.6 g

Respiratory and Mucus Syrup (Elderberry Syrup)

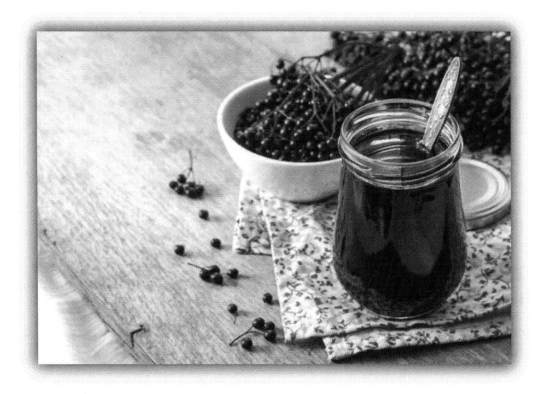

- ➢ **Preparation time:** 5 minutes
- ➢ **Cooking time:** 15 minute
- ➢ **Servings:** 2

Ingredients:

- 1 teaspoon elderberry fruit.
- 1 cup spring water.

Directions:

1. Place all ingredients in a small pan.
2. Boil for 15 minutes and remove from heat, cover and leave for another 10 minutes.
3. Strain and serve the drink.

Nutrition:

- Calories: 130
- Fat: 16 g

- Carbs: 9.5 g
- Protein: 8 g

Immune Boosting Tea

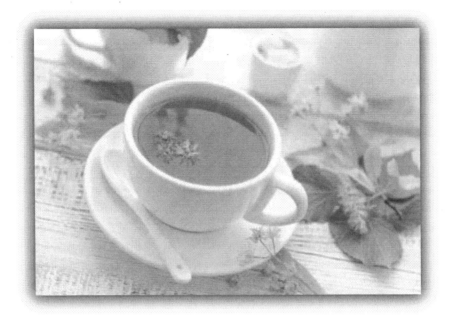

- ➢ **Preparation time:** 5 minutes
- ➢ **Cooking time:** 10 minutes
- ➢ **Servings:** 2

Ingredients:

- 1 teaspoon linden powder
- 1 teaspoon bay leaves
- 1 cup spring water

Directions:

1. Place all ingredients in a tea kettle.
2. Boil for 5 minutes and remove it from heat, cover, and leave for an additional 10 minutes.
3. Drain and serve.

Nutrition:

- Calories: 81
- Fat: 6 g
- Carbs: 4 g
- Protein: 3 g

Conclusion

Smoothies are a very easy and fun way to consume fruits and vegetables. They are simple to prepare, convenient and tasty, as well as satisfying to the eye, thanks to their vibrant colors.

The foods we eat have a huge impact on our mood, strength, energy levels, weight, concentration, immunity, longevity, and overall life. And healthy foods like smoothie ingredients are the healthiest choice there is.

Fruit and vegetable smoothies can change your life. Starting or continuing with the habit of drinking smoothies will increase your well-being by increasing the amount of fruits, vegetables, seeds, and nuts you consume. And these healthy foods will energize your mind, body, and spirit and can be one of the most powerful and best aspects of nutrition for your health.

Healthy food that is easy to prepare

Smoothies are a quick and easy way to fill your diet with nutritious foods, getting you deliciously closer to your healthy goals. And even if you're already a smoothie lover, there are endless creative combinations of flavors and a vast array of ingredients to make tasty fruit and vegetable smoothies (try a green smoothie diet, too).

Sometimes culinary inspiration is as simple as an ingredient. A flavor. A photograph. A description. An aroma. A texture.

Benefits of drinking smoothies

If by chance you've forgotten them, I want to give you a definitive rundown on the many benefits of drinking plant-based smoothies, ranging from nutritional to psychological. Here are a few of them:

- **Immune System Strengthening** - Fruits and vegetables are full of vitamins, minerals, antioxidants, phytochemicals, and other beneficial nutrients that help strengthen the immune system. Smoothies are an easy way to consume them.

- **Natural Energy Boost** - Smoothies contain fruits, high in immediate carbohydrates; therefore, they can be a big natural energy boost. Sugar is broken down by your body into glucose and released into your bloodstream as energy.

- **Healthy Weight Loss** - Smoothies are good for weight loss because they make it easy to consume adequate amounts of vitamins and minerals but maintain a calorie deficit. Many smoothies have a large amount of protein that helps satisfy hunger and prevent overeating later in the day.

- **Reduce Cholesterol** - Fruits and vegetables are rich in fiber that helps lower bad cholesterol and maintain health by lowering blood pressure. Smoothies are rich in fruit, which is just as good for lowering cholesterol as vegetables but are easier to consume because they sometimes contain a lot of liquid.

- **Cortisol Reduction** - Many smoothies contain a lot of water, which is good for keeping cortisol, the stress hormone, down. It takes your body a while to process the sugars in the fruit, and as a result, it can help you calm down.

- **Increases stamina** - Several smoothies contain large amounts of fruits and vegetables rich in vitamins and antioxidants. These help you get energy from healthy foods rather than sugars from processed foods. They also help improve your stamina in the gym, helping you in heavier sports without feeling fatigued.

- **Boosts brain power** - Fruits have been known for centuries to be great brain food, and the same goes for smoothies! They contain natural sugar that your brain needs to function well.

- **Cholesterol Decreasing** - Fruits and vegetables lower bad cholesterol, which is valuable for reducing the risk of heart disease. They contain extra nutrients than other foods, as well as more fiber, which also helps in lowering cholesterol.

- **Sense of satiety** - Fruits, especially non-watery fruits (bananas, avocados, kiwi (green), mango (yellow), papaya, contain a whole host of prebiotic substances in their fiber (unlike juices or sodas), so you won't feel hungry throughout the day.

Printed in Great Britain
by Amazon

4094850SR00097